NEW HOPE!

The supporters of megavitamin therapy believe it is the most exciting discovery of the century. Although it's young and still controversial, the authors say it promises to revolutionize treatment while reducing the cost dramatically.

Simple solutions to tough health problems are not offered, but many exciting and encouraging successes are reported in the case studies in this book.

Megavitamin Therapy

by Ruth Adams
and
Frank Murray

Larchmont Books
NEW YORK

NOTICE: This book is meant as an informational guide for the prevention of disease. For conditions of ill-health, we recommend that you see a physician, psychiatrist or other professional licensed to treat disease. These days, many medical practitioners are discovering that a strong nutritional program supports and fortifies whatever therapy they may use, as well as effectively preventing a recurrence of the illness.

Fifth printing: March 1980
Fourth printing: December, 1977
Third printing: October, 1974
Second printing: December, 1973

MEGAVITAMIN THERAPY

Copyright © 1973 by Larchmont Press

ISBN 0-915962-03-9

Printed in the United States of America.

LARCHMONT BOOKS
6 East 43rd Street
New York, N.Y. 10017

Contents

Foreword

THIS RESPONSIBLE BOOK gathers together an enormous amount of clinical and scientific data and presents it in a clear and documented way which is understandable to the average reader. The American public has become increasingly concerned with both the beneficial and deleterious effects of substances which they take into themselves or which impinge on them from their environment. The dietary pattern which predisposes individuals to the development of a number of illnesses is well described in the first chapter. I would say it is the typical diet of most of the patients I have seen with alcoholism, schizophrenia, drug abuse problems, as well as obesity and a variety of other social and medical afflictions.

In a study just concluded in industry, it was found that the accident rate amongst workers who did not eat breakfast was twice that of people who ate any kind of a breakfast. I call this the fatal All-American-Supermarket-Madison-Avenue-TV-Ad-Teen-Age-Diet, which is the diet of the average American. This is the diet which is supported by establishment nutritionists who have the nerve to make public statements that the American Supermarket provides an adequate, nourishing diet.

Most of the diseases and afflictions of mankind are now seen to be self-induced or preventable. Prevention requires an awareness of one's genetic vulnerabilities, plus essential knowledge so that one can follow a prophylactic nutritional program with a resultant decrease in susceptibility to the illnesses which are implied by one's genetic endowment. The emphasis today amongst knowledgeable people is on the actual prevention of disease. The individual who becomes sick has failed, and has brought a disease upon himself through ignorance.

Until recently, however, he was not responsible for this ignorance. The average citizen is under-educated, mis-educated and generally brainwashed into unhealthy patterns which must inevitably lead to overt illness. The physician is only brought into the picture after the horse is out of the barn. The physician himself has had little help in his own education about the importance of preventive diets and life styles. Indeed, it is only in the last two years that both the Academy of Preventive Medicine and the Academy of Orthomolecular Psychiatry have been established.

Because the average person has no contact with a physician until he has already succumbed to illness, the medical profession is very limited in what it can do to actually prevent illness. It is, therefore, up to the intelligent layman to learn all he can, not only to avoid illness but to achieve optimal health and a state of well being for himself and his family. This requires the availability of essential information with proper emphasis on decisively important concepts such as those which are presented in this basic book. The authors have provided critical information plus references for the acquisition of even more essential knowledge.

The reader should make specific notes of the illnesses which have occurred in his own family so as to become aware of his genetic vulnerabilities. Then, by means of the various tests outlined in this book, he should become acquainted with his own clinical makeup. Finally, by the study of the material in these chapters, it will become obvious that by merely changing diet and life patterns he can avoid the development of most of the illnesses and disasters which befall the uninformed.

DAVID R. HAWKINS, M.D.
Medical Director,
The North Nassau Mental Health Center
Manhasset, New York
May 17, 1973

Introduction

ORTHOMOLECULAR MEDICINE is developing rapidly and marks a major shift in the evolution of medicine and psychiatry. Between 1930 and 1940 the vitamin decade left us enriched food and a vast amount of unused information. The next decade of antibiotics helped conquer many of our serious infections but did not tell us why only some were infected. The Fifties introduced the wonder drugs (cortisone and ACTH), which still have a useful role. The Sixties introduced the tranquilizer and anti-depressant era. The Seventies will mark the orthomolecular era.

At last major attention is given to the role of diet and special nutrients in maintaining health. At last information painfully gained over the past 50 years is being applied on a large scale. We know that too little protein and too much refined carbohydrates (alcohol, sugar, white flour) are behind the illness and misery suffered by millions of people. We know that people are biochemically different and that some will require many times the recommended daily doses of vitamins and minerals. All of this is the subject matter of orthomolecular medicine.

This is the subject matter of this well-written, well-researched book. It is one of the first books on orthomolecular medicine for everyone. It is an essential book for everyone who values his own mental and physical health and that of his family and community. For the explosive pandemic of ill health, addiction and mental disease will not be contained until the principles of orthomolecular medicine are widely understood and practiced.

A. HOFFER, M.D., PH.D.
Saskatoon, Saskatchewan, Canada
President, The Huxley Institute for
   Biosocial Research,
New York, N. Y.
May 2, 1973

CHAPTER 1

"I Am
a Cured
Alcoholic"

"I AM A cured alcoholic," said a letter which came to us recently. "A brother died of alcoholism in his mid-50's. An alcoholic sister died of heart complications in her mid-50's. All of us were brought up in the same home, with the same inheritance in terms of susceptibility to disease—*and with the same eating patterns.*

"I stress the eating patterns, along with patterns of susceptibility to disease. Everyone knows that diseases like diabetes 'run in families.' If you have a diabetic mother, you're more likely to get the disease than if you don't. If both parents are diabetic, you're much more likely to get the disease.

"But somehow doctors in general diagnose diseases such as diabetes without ever inquiring about events in the patient's life, aside from inherited genes, which might have brought on the disease. It is my belief that alcoholism—and probably drug addiction—are the result of inherited patterns of susceptibility, *com-*

*bined with patterns of eating that are established
very early in life.*

"My parents were opposed to drinking. Liquor
(even beer or wine) was unknown in our home.
But our patterns of living and eating predisposed
each of the children in that family to a life of alcoholism or some other form of addiction. I am
certain of it. We never—or almost never—ate breakfast. On Saturdays, Sundays and holidays some of
us had breakfast—a breakfast that was always cereal,
sugar, pancakes loaded with carbohydrates, or waf-
fles with maple syrup. But on weekdays, we went off
to school (and my father to work) with no breakfast.
Lunch was sketchy. If we were at the school cafe-
teria, we invariably chose foods that were mostly
high carbohydrate: potatoes, pasta, desserts, sweet
rolls. No one had ever told us not to eat such things.

"Dinner was the only fairly well-planned meal of
the day, and it was always badly conceived in terms
of what we now know is good, sound nutritional
practice. Meat and potatoes were the usual fare at
dinner. None of us ever drank milk. Desserts were
not only served at every meal, but also candy and
cookies were always available at any time of the day.
We ate lots of this kind of food.

"My mother was a coffee addict. She ate almost
nothing all day, but she drank coffee continuously
from early morning until late at night. She suffered
from many infectious diseases, was tired and complaining all the time, had migraine headaches which
kept her in bed, vomiting, for several days every
two weeks or so. The headaches were there when

she awakened in the morning. The best therapy, she felt, was coffee—another cup every hour or so and she would eventually be able to get out of bed and stagger about doing her housework until the next headache appeared.

"As we youngsters grew up and went off to college, we discovered liquor. And all three of us found that this one substance, taken often enough throughout the day, could ease the jitters in our stomachs, cure fatigue (we thought), and bring us a marvelous feeling of well-being and relaxation. And so for all those years we continued to slight breakfast, ate no lunch or a skimpy one at best, then relaxed with a big dinner and plenty of booze. If drugs other than alcohol had been in general circulation at that time, I'm sure we would have been 'hooked' on all of them, just as we were hooked on alcohol and tobacco.

"Looking back on those difficult years, I cannot remember a day when I did not suffer from many varieties of weakness, dizziness, faintness, hunger and sometimes rather frightening hallucinations which preceded headaches. When I was tired and overworked, all the symptoms were worse. Vacations and days when I could rest they all but disappeared, so it was comforting that, in my early 20's, I had at last found two substances which could temporarily relieve most of the distressing symptoms—cigarettes and alcohol. Of course, the symptoms always returned by noon the next day. For years I lit a cigarette as soon as I got up every morning. It made me dizzy, but it quieted the butterflies in my stomach. Coffee and cigarettes got me through the morning.

"By the time I was 30, I had to have a big chocolate bar every morning about 10 and a dose of some kind of sugary goody by 4 in the afternoon, just to keep going. No breakfast and a meager lunch continued to be the rule. By five o'clock, the only thing that could possibly keep me going through the evening was a drink or two—or three. During one period of great stress, I found that I was drinking my lunch and drinking all afternoon and evening as well. Soon a drink was essential to get me started in the morning; my hands trembled uncontrollably without it. I still ate no breakfast, for the drink took the place of it.

"My brother and sister were pursuing this same path. My brother had reached the same point that I had—he was drinking all day, too. In addition to the all-day drinking, he often went to evening parties, where there was lots more drinking. I never became drunk, never passed out, never had a hangover, as such. But I *had* to have booze or I simply could not get through the day. I had a vague idea that it was harming me, but it was impossible for me to do without it. When I had to go on trips, or to visit in someone's home where liquor was unavailable, I took some along. On business trips I often had to retire to the bathroom, get out my bottle and have a drink every hour or so. Without it I would have passed out or become so nervous and jittery that I couldn't have conducted any business.

"Eventually, when I was well on my way to alcoholism, I began to work in a medical library, where it was my job to sort and catalog all the publications that came in. I began to read about alcoholism; I began to read about diet. I had access to all the literature I needed on both subjects, and so I began to change my way of eating. I ate eggs for breakfast, and I was astonished at the stability and feeling of well being this single item of food brought me. I switched to two eggs with bacon or ham, and I began to cut down on coffee. The results were remarkable. I could get along without a drink at mid-morning. And I forced myself to eat a high-protein lunch —lots of meat, cheese, milk. I found that I could get through the afternoon without a drink—if I had a 4 o'clock snack of cheese, peanuts or some other high-protein food.

"Meanwhile, I was reading the vast amounts of literature then becoming available on smoking and the health disasters it can bring. I decided to stop smoking, convinced that I would black out, would collapse from nervousness and tension, but determined to try. It was easy. There was hardly any nervousness or other withdrawal symptoms. I was cured of my addiction to nicotine!

"During this time I found occasional articles on other aspects of addiction, including one world-shaking report of a doctor who cured confirmed alcoholics by injecting high-protein meals and large doses of vitamins into their stomachs! Unbelievable, I thought. It is a well-known scientific fact that alcoholism is a psychological thing, an inherited thing! How can you cure it with food and vitamins?

But why not try?

"I ordered some vitamins and took them—the B Complex and vitamin C especially—in extremely large quantities. I increased the protein content of my diet until I was eating up to 125 grams of protein a day—cheese and high-protein bread, along with my bacon and eggs for breakfast. Cheese, meat and high-protein bread for lunch. Dinner consisted of almost nothing but high-protein foods—meat, fish, poultry, eggs, cheese—and almost no carbohydrates. Snacks were always high-protein. The vitamins and the high-protein meals became a way of life. *And I found that I no longer had the almost-constant craving for alcohol.* The only time of day when drinking had the slightest attraction for me was just before dinner, when I was most fatigued, most hungry.

I experimented. Some days I had a highball or a cocktail before dinner. Other days I did not. There didn't seem to be much difference in the way I felt with or without liquor. So why drink? If dinner were delayed, I found myself wishing for a drink. If it was on the table when I got home, I had no wish for a drink. At parties I found myself taking ginger ale or tomato juice and carrying it around as if it contained a shot or two of booze. Or I would put a jigger of liquor in it and nurse the glass all evening. Nobody but me knew the difference. I also refused all invitations to cocktail parties as such, since I knew that, at such a party, there would inevitably be lots of liquor and almost no food. I still do not go to cocktail parties. If, in my work, I have to attend one, I eat an entire high-protein dinner before I go. Thus, I feel no need for a drink, even when everyone around me is drinking.

"I call myself a cured alcoholic. I know that experts in this field declare positively that there is no such thing—that the true alcoholic can never take a drink again if he wants to remain sober. So, perhaps, I am not a true alcoholic. If the experts had known me 25 years ago, when I was living on booze with almost no food at all, I think they would have diagnosed me as an alcoholic. In any case, there may be many others just like me who *can* overcome their craving for alcohol and, hopefully, cigarettes as well, by maintaining the kind of dietary program I maintain. I don't know. But I think they should be given the chance to hear about it so they can try it for themselves. I hope that you will be able to use this information to inform them."

We also think that such a story should be told so that readers who may have the same general kind of background may possibly benefit from it. The success of this individual in treating the craving for alcohol and nicotine, with diet and diet supplements, seems to confirm the evidence which we had already assembled for this book. And, as we will see in later chapters, there is a definite correlation between alcoholism, drug addiction and mental illness—and low blood sugar. Many of today's young people— whose non-nourishing diets and addiction to coffee and cigarettes are already well known—are turning away from hard drugs. And where are they turning? To alcohol!

CHAPTER 2

Alcohol—a Major Drug Problem

ACCORDING TO *The New York Times* for March 9, 1972, alcohol addiction warps some 9,000,000 lives in the United States, costs about $15 billion annually, causes directly or indirectly almost half of all arrests in this country. Heavy drinkers shorten their life-span by 10 to 12 years and cause incalculable grief to their unfortunate families.

"There is a large, profitable and flourishing industry built on liquor in this country, and there is no reason why its resources should not be tapped for additional funds necessary to treat problem alcoholics, to do research on prevention and cure, and to educate the public that alcohol abuse is in a class with many other forms of drug abuse," the *Times* stated.

"Alcohol is a *factor* in at least half the motor vehicle fatalities each year," stated James P. Kielty, Road Safety Supervisor, Public Information Department, National Safety Council, Chicago, Ill. "During 1972, a total of 56,300 persons died in traffic accidents nationwide. Therefore, alcohol was a factor in about 30,000 of these deaths. I can't give an estimate of the property loss, but the cost of *all* traffic accidents during 1972 was $17.5 billion," Mr. Kielty said in a letter to us on February 12, 1973. "This included fatal and non-fatal as well as property damage."

A University of Michigan survey turned up the fact that of 72 persons judged responsible for fatal accidents, half were alcoholics or pre-alcoholics. *Among them they had been responsible for 87 deaths in a period of three years.*

"Drinking (of alcohol or many other drugs) removes inhibitions," said a British physician in a letter to the *British Medical Journal.* "Drinking without inhibitions causes accidents. Statistics of conviction for drunken driving or relating road accidents to intoxication barely skim the surface of the problem. They confuse the issue and divert attention from the real issue, the killer which is 'drinking and driving.' "

James P. Kielty said that the National Safety Council does not have statistics on how many people are arrested in the United States each year for drunk driving. However, it is estimated that there are more than 100 million licensed drivers who can be considered social drinkers—in other words, about one-half the population. Approximately another nine million drivers with and without driver licenses can be considered abusive drinkers, he said.

"The federal government, under provisions of the Highway Safety Act of 1966, requires that all states take three steps to get drunk drivers off the roads. These include: providing for 'implied consent' laws, a blood-alcohol content of 0.10 per cent to determine intoxication, and 'tests on fatals,' a blood-alcohol test on accident victims and drivers surviving accidents fatal to others.

"All states and the District of Columbia," Mr. Kielty continued, "have 'implied consent' laws on the books, most have the 0.10 law, and about 20 states have the 'tests on fatals' provision."

Added Mr. Kielty: "The chances of being ar-

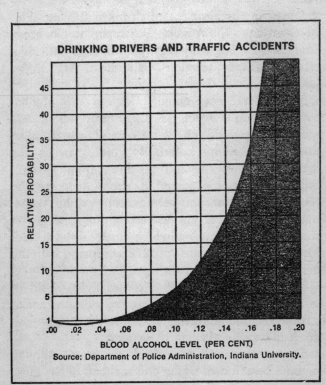

DRINKING DRIVERS AND TRAFFIC ACCIDENTS

RELATIVE PROBABILITY

BLOOD ALCOHOL LEVEL (PER CENT)

Source: Department of Police Administration, Indiana University.

rested for driving while intoxicated have been estimated at one in 2,000. The average police officer only makes two drunk-driver arrests each year. The U. S. Department of Transportation figures for 1968 show that only 5 per cent—one in 20 drivers—initially charged with drunken driving were ever convicted of the offense."

Although there are no statistics on the percentage increase of drunken drivers within, say, the past 10 years, there is a definite increase in attention being paid to the problem of drunken driving. This stemmed from the August 1968 report to Congress, "Alcohol and Highway Safety," from the then Secretary of Transportation Alan Boyd, Mr. Kielty said.

The federal government, through the Alcohol Safety Action Project, is distributing about $84 million among 35 cities to rehabilitate drunken drivers, Mr. Kielty noted. By zeroing in on the drunken driver, the toll resulting from alcohol-related deaths is expected to drop. According to former U. S. Transportation Secretary John Volpe, the proof of the current ASAP program success was shown by New Orleans, which cut fatalities in half for the first three months of 1972, compared with the first three months of 1971, Mr. Kielty said.

On September 14, 1972, Howard Pyle, president of the National Safety Council, urged states not to pass legislation allowing 18-year-olds to buy and drink all types of alcoholic beverages.

"Younger persons who drink are more likely to become involved in traffic crashes than older, more experienced drinking drivers—even though the young persons may have fairly low blood-alcohol concentrations," Governor Pyle said. "Unfortunately," he added, "18-year-olds are still learning the driving task at the same time they are learning how to drink. The results are proving to be tragic."

In January 1973, Governor Pyle asked the nation's brewers and distillers to label alcoholic beverage containers with a cautionary statement saying that excessive drinking will impair driving ability.

"Although research shows the majority of the public is aware of the potential hazards of drinking and driving, too many (people) who drink still do not make adequate use of this knowledge," Governor Pyle said in *The New York Times,* January 31, 1973.

He agreed that chronic alcoholics would probably pay little attention to the warning. "But," he said, "the alcoholic beverage industry would perform a public service for the responsible, well-meaning consumers of its product," the *Times* said.

The National Safety Council states that an individual who continues to drink more rapidly than the alcohol is eliminated from his body generally goes through the following stages: sobriety, elation, excitement, confusion, stupor, unconsciousness . . . death.

A driver with a blood-alcohol level of 0.15 per cent has a 25 times greater chance of *causing* a traffic accident than he would if he were not drinking, the Council reports. Increased accident causation is noticeable at 0.04 per cent, and probability is at least six times as great at 0.10 per cent. The risk factor for pedestrians is indicated to be similar.

The person involved in an auto accident following drinking may be characterized as belonging to one of three groups, according to the National Safety Council. These are: 1) the heavy drinker with aggressive behavior; 2) the chronic alcoholic; and 3) the social drinker. The proportion of motor vehicle accidents in the United States attributable to persons in these three groups is not presently known, but there is increasing evidence to indicate that persons suffering from chronic alcoholism, while representing a small percentage of the drivers, are responsible for a disproportionately large percentage of accidents after drinking.

"Studies indicate that 20 per cent of males and almost 9 per cent of the females in home accidents had been drinking," the Council said. "Such accidents included falling asleep with lighted cigarettes, poisonings and drownings."

"Sociologists say of alcoholism among housewives the same thing they say about murder among the middle-class—there is a lot more of it than is ever suspected or discovered," reports the *New York Post*, April 2, 1973. J. W. Bedell, Professor and Chairman of the Department of Sociology, California State University, Fullerton, said that many alcoholic housewives are "9 a.m. to 3 p.m. drinkers", who drink only during school hours when they are alone at home. Bedell, who has received a new National Science Foundation grant to continue his studies of alcoholic housewives, said that a number of them, when they begin to fear that their drinking has been noticed by neighbors, persuade their husbands to move to a new town and get a new job, the *Post* said. "If the husband is reluctant, the wife may go so far as to get a divorce so she can live among new neighbors," Bedell added.

Continued the *Post:* "Many alcoholic women keep their secret from everybody except their husbands and doctors, and the doctors usually find out only while treating them for some condition such as obesity, high blood pressure or depression. Most of the alcoholic women he interviews tell him they have friends who also drink too much."

Bedell said that some psychologists have theorized that many alcoholic women grew up in homes where the fathers adjusted "orally" to day-to-day tensions.

ALCOHOLIC BEVERAGES	Alcohol Content	BLOOD ALCOHOL LEVELS One Drink*					
		NORMAL MEASURE	Alcohol Content	Body Weight in Lbs.			
				100	140	180	220
Beer	4%	12-oz. Bottle	(Oz.) .48	.04	% .03	.02	.02
Wine	12%	3-oz. Glass	.36	.03	.03	.02	.02
Liqueur	40%	1-oz. Glass	.40	.03	.03	.02	.02
Distilled Spirits	45%	1-oz. Glass	.45	.04	.03	.02	.02
Mixed Drinks	30%	3½-oz. Glass	1.05	.08	.06	.04	.04

* This constitutes estimated potential blood alcohol levels that can be achieved within a normal drinking period.

Source: National Safety Council

These were habits associated with their mouths—biting fingernails, gnawing the knuckles, working the jaw muscles and chewing the lower lip.

"Two other examples," Bedell said, "are smoking and excessive drinking."

Alcoholism is also a serious problem in industry, the Council said. Hangovers interfere with the safe operation of machinery, resulting in accidents, even when the employee isn't actually under the influence on the job.

"Studies indicate that employees who are alcoholics have more than twice as many on-the-job accidents—and at least 10 times as many off-the-job accidents—as non-drinkers," the National Safety Council stated.

Alcohol (ethyl alcohol) is a mood-changing drug like cocaine, heroin, barbiturates, amphetamines, etc. Alcohol is a depressant that acts as an anesthetic on the central nervous system. It is absorbed unchanged in the stomach and small intestine and is disseminated by the blood to all parts of the body, including the brain.

According to the National Safety Council, blood-alcohol concentration in the body is related to:

1) Body weight.

2) The amount of alcohol consumed.

3) The length of time since drinking began.

4) The length of time since the last drink.

5) The quantity and kind of food in the stomach at the time of drinking.

"About 90 to 95 per cent of the alcohol is metabolized into carbon dioxide and water," the Council said. "The other 5 to 10 per cent is excreted through the lungs and kidneys. Black coffee, cold showers and physical exercise may seem to make the drinker more alert, but they do *not* accelerate the elimination of alcohol from the body.

"In the brain, alcohol first depresses the area of higher functions, which includes judgment and social restraint. Next, it attacks the simple motor functions, reaction time and vision. Balance, co-ordination and sensory perception are the next faculties to be impaired," the Council said.

It is estimated that eight out of 10 men over 21 and two out of three women over 21 drink alcoholic beverages. And, as we reported earlier, there are some nine million alcoholics in the United States.

"Alcoholism," states the National Council on Alcoholism, Inc., 2 Park Ave., New York, N. Y. 10016, "has been called the most serious drug problem, in terms of number of victims and cost to society, physical damage to the body and its organs, and the large number of fatalities resulting from withdrawal symptoms.

"Alcoholism ranks among the major national health threats, along with cancer, mental illness and heart disease. Yet the U. S. Department of Health, Education and Welfare has termed alcoholism this country's most neglected disease."

We have already seen the tragic consequences of alcoholism and traffic accidents. The National Council on Alcoholism provides some additional alarming statistics:

1) Alcoholism is a complex, progressive illness.

Alcoholics are sick, just as people suffering from heart disease or cancer are sick. If not treated, alcoholism ends in permanent mental damage, physical incapacity or early death.

2) The average alcoholic is a man or woman in the middle 30's with a good job, a good home, and a family. Less than 5 per cent of alcoholics are found on Skid Row.

3) Some 6.5 million employed workers are alcoholics.

4) An estimated 200,000 Federal-civilian employees suffer from alcoholism. Benefits from Federal employee alcoholism programs are projected to $1.25 billion over five years, or $17 saved for every $1 spent.

5) 40 per cent of all male admissions to state mental hospitals suffer from alcoholism.

6) Alcoholism accounts—directly or indirectly—for 40 per cent of the problems brought to family courts.

7) 31 per cent of those who take their own lives are alcoholics. Their suicide rate is 58 times that of non-alcoholics.

"Figures for alcoholism in the drinking population have remained constant since 1940, that is about 6 per cent of those who choose to drink alcoholic beverages on a regular basis seem to develop alcoholism," stated Mr. Yvelin Gardner, Assistant to the Executive Director, National Council on Alcoholism, in a letter to us. "As the adult population increases, the drinking population has increased, and, although numerically there are more alcoholics than before, they represent the same per cent of total drinkers.

"Alcoholism seems to develop in people who drink at the crucial ages between 35 and 50, when they are at the peak of productivity and responsibility. There is no particular occupation which has indicated any higher incidence of alcoholism than any other," Mr. Gardner continued. "Newspaper writers, bartenders, advertising men, etc., have claimed to have more alcoholics than others. But every profession or trade or labor field seems to have about the same potential for alcoholism as any other."

Mr. Gardner added that, although the major causes of alcoholism are still to be determined, it is generally agreed that there is a metabolic dysfunction which develops in some people after varying years of drinking, which causes loss of control so that such people cannot take one drink with impunity. "We have not located as yet the physical area in the body which develops this function, but much research is being done to discover it," Mr. Gardner said.

While doctors, psychiatrists, non-profit organizations and others wrestle with the causes and treatment of alcoholism, we hope to show in this book that there is possibly another way to deal with this human tragedy—through diet and nutrition.

CHAPTER 3

Alcoholism— an Addiction?

THE AMERICAN HOSPITAL ASSOCIATION declared recently that 25 to 30 per cent of all adult medical-surgical patients in metropolitan hospitals, regardless of diagnosis, were found to be suffering from alcoholism. Fifty per cent of all fractures result from drunkenness, the Association added.

Alcohol has the qualities of inducing tolerance and withdrawal symptoms—two qualities which are associated with physiological dependence or addiction. This happens after a varying, but usually long preliminary period of heavy social drinking. However, we do not as yet know why one out of every 15 adult U. S. drinkers ends up as an alcoholic. Why don't the other 14?

Nobody knows the answer to this basic question, and surprisingly little is being done to find out, considering the disease's prevalence. For example, why don't doctors know more about alcoholism and its treatment? In 1956, Dr. Marvin Block, a professor of medicine, worked out a curriculum on alcoholism for medical colleges. He sent copies to each medical school in the country, and to each department head.

A dozen years later, no medical school was giving any of the recommended courses.

In February 1971, *Medical World News* reported that, for the 900,000 cancer patients in this country, $70 million are being collected in fund drives. For cerebral palsy, with 100,000 victims, almost $39 million dollars are taken in yearly. For muscular dystrophy, with 200,000 victims, almost $10 million are channeled to help these unfortunates. For alcoholism, with its previously reported nine million sufferers, a mere $2 million are given annually to help in treatment.

Statistics show that the average untreated alcoholic's life-span is shortened by 12 years, yet most cases of alcoholism in the United States fail to get adequate medical attention. Early symptoms often go unrecognized. And alcoholism still suffers from the effects of social and moral prejudices which retard its recognition as an illness and, therefore, discourage urgently needed professional treatment.

If your answer is "yes" to any of the following key questions, prepared by the National Council on Alcoholism, you have some of the symptoms that *may* indicate incipient alcoholism:

1) Difficult to get along with when drinking.
2) Drink because you are depressed.
3) Drink to calm your nerves.
4) Drink until you are often "dead drunk."
5) Can't remember parts of some episodes.
6) Hide liquor.
7) Lie about your drinking.
8) Neglect to eat when you are drinking.

9) Neglect your family or job when you are drinking.

If you suspect that you may be slowly drifting into alcoholism, by all means seek expert advice right away. There may be a local Alcoholics Anonymous chapter close to your home. If you wish, you can contact the National Council on Alcoholism, whose address has already been given, or Alcoholics Anonymous World Services, Inc., Box 459, Grand Central Station, New York, N. Y. 10017. If you are lucky enough not to have an alcohol problem, why not make a donation to either or both of the above-named, worthwhile organizations.

The precise roles of the physical predisposition and psychological factors and the combination of psychology, predisposition and cultural availability of alcohol in the genesis of alcoholism are not known. It is not impossible that a lab test for susceptibility to alcoholism could be found. Research on these many variables in alcoholism is much needed and is a goal of the National Council on Alcoholism.

Chemical aspects of alcoholism provide an exciting subject for future study. Fortunately, however, effective and tested methods of rehabilitation are already available and have proven highly successful in thousands and thousands of cases. But the key to rehabilitation for today's alcoholic rests largely in the hands of his family and friends. It is *they* who must first realize how impossible it is for an alcoholic to fight against his addiction without competent professional help. They must see to it that he gets such help as easily as possible.

Alcoholics Anonymous is doing an outstanding job in this area. It is an informal society of an estimated 475,000 men and women who have recovered from alcoholism; about one-fourth of the membership are women. There are chapters in many countries throughout the world, in Canada and the United States, in public and private hospitals, rest homes and convalescent facilities, as well as in penal institutions. A.A. works closely with administrators and members in providing counseling, literature and other services. Check your telephone directory to see if there is an A.A. chapter near you.

A.A., incidentally, evolved from the experience of two men, Bill W., a former New York stockbroker, and Dr. Bob S., an Akron, Ohio surgeon. A.A.'s tradition has always been never to reveal the true name of any member.

"Bill," the Association stated, "whose compulsive drinking had caused him to be declared a hopeless drunkard, achieved sobriety in December 1934, following an unusual spiritual experience. The following spring, he was able to help free Dr. Bob from his alcoholic compulsion.

"The two men noted that their own desire to drink disappeared when they tried to share their recovery experience with other alcoholics," the A.A. continued. "The chain reaction resulting from this discovery has been responsible for the consistent growth of the movement. Dr. Bob died in 1950. Bill W. continued to be active in the movement as a writer and adviser." Regrettably, Bill has since passed away.

Like many diseases that get worse by degrees, alcoholism is difficult to spot but easiest to treat in its early stages. The time that separates heavy drinking from alcoholism is a thin one, notes the National Council on Alcoholism. Yet the physician, who should be an expert in the detection of all disease, is often poorly equipped by his early training to detect the early signs.

A high proportion of alcoholics are well-off in a financial way, and many hold high-paying jobs, which they are gradually forced to neglect as their disease gets worse—unless they are among the lucky few who now receive treatment.

Many alcoholics, the NCA states, have a lot of "strength of character," yet they become alcoholics. Why? Alcoholics have in common only the fact that their daily intake of the drug—alcohol—exceeds their body's ability to handle it effectively.

All of us who drink socially—even if we are quite moderate drinkers—could be prone to the disease of alcoholism, the NCA points out. For this reason, if for no other, we must all try to help establish a climate of public opinion which recognizes alcoholism for what it is—a disease—and to support the establishment of expanded research and treatment facilities.

Dr. Milton Halpern, New York City's Chief Medical Examiner, said that alcoholism was more frequently associated with homicide than were drugs, according to the May 23, 1973 issue of the *New York Post*. Dr. Halpern, who was addressing an all-day physicians' conference on alcoholism at the New York University Medical Center, added that there were more alcoholics than drug addicts in the city.

Dr. Halpern is quoted as saying that about 50 per cent of violent deaths in New York City, as well as in the U.S. as a whole, are associated with alcohol. "And some natural deaths are hastened by alcohol," he said.

"The stigma attached to the disease of alcoholism is still so great that many doctors find it 'convenient' to omit any mention of it when making out death certificates," Halpern said. "They claim to be protecting the families. Actually, they are perpetuating the stigma."

Speaking at the same conference, Dr. Robert J. Campbell, Associate Director, Psychiatry Dept., St. Vincent's Hospital, New York, noted that alcoholism was becoming more of a problem among the young. He added that 65 per cent of those between 22 and 25 drank regularly.

In a discussion of whether alcoholism is actually a disease, *American Medical News* presents this sentence by a New Orleans doctor: "Why certain individuals are able to sustain themselves without the use of alcohol, or, for that matter, the physician-prescribed tranquilizers, is a question that we are not yet able to answer."

We suggest that the reason is simply that this gentleman and many other professionals have not looked at all the facts. Certainly the evidence shows clearly that individuals who become alcoholics are born with certain biological or metabolic characteristics which are quite different from those who never feel any need for alcohol. And obviously, from all the evidence, this biological difference has something to do with the body's use of carbohydrates.

Would anyone doubt that diabetes is a disease? Does not alcoholism show many of the same symptoms as diabetes? Would any of us insist that the diabetic go without treatment, since we do not know how he becomes diabetic? And isn't it likely that the same general kind of nutritive treatment will benefit the alcoholic as it does the diabetic?

Some experts in this field believe—or used to believe—that alcoholism should not be called an addiction, in the same sense that drug addiction is. An experiment conducted in 1964 seems to prove the opposite. Ten formerly alcoholic volunteers in a prison were given measured amounts of alcohol under strict supervision by Dr. Jack Mendelson of Harvard University.

Every four hours, all day long, a new drink appeared while the prisoners were free to enjoy themselves in the recreation room. By the time they were drinking a full quart plus eight ounces of whisky daily, the experiment was terminated and the alcoholics were given no more alcohol. Almost immediately they went into typical withdrawal symptoms —the bodily and mental anguish which occurs when addicts are withdrawn from their drug, no matter what drug that may be.

The men begged and whimpered for their drinks. Then they began to hallucinate. These were men who had shown no signs of intoxication during the entire experiment. Their hearts worked harder when they were drinking, their pulse rates increased 30 per cent, and, finally, up to 70 per cent. It was found that, during heavy drinking, the body retains uric acid, the substance that causes gout. It also turns the urine alkaline, which makes the drinker more susceptible to urinary infections.

The September 1, 1972 issue of *Science* printed an article on laboratory rats kept on "an intermittent food schedule." With alcohol available instead of drinking water, the animals drank the alcohol. When it was taken away and water was substituted, they had all the symptoms of physical addiction and dependence, including convulsions and death.

Can you inherit the tendency to alcoholism? Apparently you can. A 1972 survey by Dr. M. A. Schuckit convinced him so thoroughly that he said that he would never touch liquor if he had any close relative who was an alcoholic. He studied almost 100 people—half of whom had a real parent who was alcoholic, but who were brought up by foster parents who were not alcoholic. The other group had no alcoholism in their immediate families, but were raised by foster parents who were alcoholic. Of the 23 alcoholics, 65 per cent had a real parent who was an alcoholic but only 19 per cent of the non-alcoholics had a real parent who was.

"Having an alcoholic's genes is more important than being raised by one," said Dr. Schuckit.

Although it would be infinitely harder to uncover the relationship, is it not possible that the genes do not necessarily predict alcoholism for any individual, but may simply give him such a constitution that he may succumb to alcoholism, or overweight, diabetes, drug addiction, or any of the disorders that are related to an individual's inability to handle carbohydrate? If, for example, he is raised in some location where he cannot get alcohol, wouldn't he be as likely to turn into a sugar-addict? Wouldn't he be as likely to turn to drugs such as heroin and/ or barbiturates, amphetamines, etc., if he could get them?

If addiction springs from the same metabolic source, regardless of what one is addicted to, couldn't he simply become addicted to coffee or soft drinks as many people are? The swings in blood sugar levels resulting from heavy coffee consumption cause one to "need" coffee or "another coke" at those times when blood sugar plunges rapidly down and the inevitable jitters come on.

A genetic and biochemical deficiency could be the reason some persons become alcoholics while others do not, stated Dr. Stanley Gitlow, president of the American Medical Society on Alcoholism, and Professor of Medicine, Mt. Sinai School of Medicine, New York. His remarks, reported by the *New York Post*, September 12, 1972, were made at an AMSA meeting at the Georgia Mental Health Institute, Atlanta.

He said that the idea that there is an "addictive personality" is slowly being dispelled and that "We are getting away from looking for psychological or moral reasons to explain alcoholism."

Dr. Gitlow added that more than 80 per cent of the alcoholics he has seen have had a blood relative who also was an alcoholic, suggesting that there may be a hereditary cause for the problem.

In a recent issue of *Medical World News*, Dr. Jack A. Mendelson, mentioned earlier in this chapter, stated that "there is no data that would prove a gene-related basis for alcoholism, and we may find that it is not so much what the alcoholic brings into the world but the way in which he or she learns to adapt to life's stresses and situations that cause alcoholism."

But, Dr. Mendelson, what is a more stressful situation than the inability to get enough of the essential nutrients to satisfy your individual needs along with constant exposure to one agent—refined white sugar—which deranges one of the most important of the body's regulatory systems—the blood sugar level?

Dr. Marvin A. Block, who attended the same symposium, said: "Drug abuse, of which alcoholism is the most common, presents a vast problem in prevention through education and communications. The alcoholic particularly has such a low discomfort threshold that he can't take the slightest annoyance and wants relief immediately. I am afraid that what I see in this country is a population largely dependent on drugs of all kinds, of which alcohol is the most readily available, and gives the greatest desired effect for the money. . . . If we could cure the whole generation of alcoholics today, we would be nowhere from a public health viewpoint unless we prevent a new, huge generation of alcoholics from replacing them."

What are some of the symptoms of alcoholism which a doctor can diagnose, although the patient insists he is not an alcoholic? Dr. Frank A. Seixas listed the following symptoms: rapid heart beat, some kind of high blood pressure, cirrhosis of the liver and hemorrhoids that may accompany it, gastritis, gout, any disease of the myocardium (the muscular tissue of the heart), any kind of anemia, and many different mouth symptoms.

Asked whether there is cross-dependency between alcohol and other drugs, Dr. Seixas said: "Both the sedatives and the narcotic drugs are depressants of the central nervous system. Cross-dependency between the sedatives, which include alcohol, paraldehyde, the barbiturates and the so-called minor tranquilizers, is very great. Individuals acquire tolerance to all the sedatives in a similar manner and require larger doses to get the same effect."

Many respected researchers have shown the cause and the treatment of alcoholism, but this research has often fallen on deaf ears. For quite some time alcoholism has been treated by diet—the same high-protein, low-carbohydrate diet with frequent meals which keeps blood sugar levels on an even keel. Records of this successful treatment for alcoholism are available in a very fine book, *Body, Mind and Sugar*, by E. M. Abrahamson and E. W. Pezet. It was published in 1951 by Holt, Rinehart and Winston, New York, in hardcover, and more recently in paperback by Pyramid Books, New York.

In another important book, *Dr. Atkins' Diet Revolution,* by Robert C. Atkins, M.D., published recently by David McKay Co., New York, Dr. Atkins has this to say: "I really cannot recommend adding sugar or sweets at any point in your (dieting) regime. I'm not talking about adding a little fruit, berries, melons, particularly. I'm talking about not adding ordinary candies, cookies, cakes, pies, rich desserts.

"The reason," he goes on, "is that such sweets are to people with a disturbed carbohydrate metabolism what alcohol is to an alcoholic, heroin to a drug addict, a pack of cigarettes to an ex-smoker, Vegas to a gambler. The safest move is to stay away from such sweets entirely. It may be that you can't take just a little; your illness doesn't permit it."

A New York physician cures alcoholics—even those with the DT's or delirium tremens—by making an opening in their stomachs and inserting a tube through which he feeds them a high-protein liquid food, plus all the vitamins and minerals.

Dr. Frank S. Butler, whose treatment was described in the *Journal of the American Geriatrics Society* for September 1967, said that he must operate on his patients because they are so dependent on alcohol and so little accustomed to eating nourishing diets that they cannot feed themselves consistently with this preparation. But, as soon as the matter is taken out of their hands and they are literally forced to be well fed, whether they want to be or not, their health improves at once and they have no difficulty in changing their usual drinking habits.

About the same time, Dr. Roger J. Williams and his associates at the University of Texas conducted experiments in which mice were made alcoholic by giving them inadequate diets and making either alcohol or water available for drinking. This resulted in producing alcoholism in about the same proportion of mice as there are people afflicted with alcoholism, which Dr. Williams interpreted to indicate that individual mice, like individual humans, have varying needs for nutrients. If these needs are satisfied by the individual's diet, he does not "take to alcohol," but can drink or not drink as he wishes, without becoming addicted. Dr. Williams could also "cure" his alcoholic mice by giving them diets high enough in protein, vitamins and minerals to meet their nutritional needs.

On the other hand, if the diet is not providing for those extra nutrients the individual desperately needs, he will try to quiet his quivering nerves and raise his sagging self-confidence by drinking alcohol to excess. The more he drinks, the more badly nourished he becomes, for alcohol contains nothing but calories—hence, nothing nourishing. The alcoholic, through no fault of his own, is thus led into a vicious circle which eventually results in his death—usually from malnutrition.

Dr. Frank S. Butler said: "Alcoholism can be controlled with a diet high in protein and rich in vitamins, especially vitamin B. Since the alcoholic cannot be expected to accept a change in diet, he must be fed involuntarily."

Dr. Williams has proved successfully that alcoholism can be induced by a diet that does not meet individual needs and can be "cured" by a diet which does. And Dr. Abrahamson showed that an excellent high-protein diet, taken at frequent intervals during the day, can provide enough of all nutrients to enable the alcoholic to climb back on the wagon permanently and stay there, as long as he adheres to the high-protein diet.

Continued Dr. Butler: "Alcoholism is a nutritional disease, as are obesity and diabetes. The compulsion to drink usually cannot be prevented—again, not unlike the desires of those who are overweight or diabetic. On the other hand, control can be effected to prevent the end-result of the inevitable deficiencies."

Dr. Butler knows the symptoms of alcoholism well. He tells us that the alcoholic is powerless to control his drinking, that he progresses to a debilitated condition by rejecting food, except for alcohol, so that the symptoms increase, the liver is affected and, finally, there is malnutrition and vitamin deficiency, which result in "irreversible and inevitable end-results."

He tells us that all the arguments in the field of medicine, psychology and sociology have brought no solutions. He goes on to say, "The physiology of the body demands essential nutrition in the form of carbohydrates, fats, proteins and vitamins. Any of these elements of diet if ingested to the exclusion of the others results in an unbalanced fuel intake. . . . Alcohol is an easily absorbed, rapidly utilized source of energy in the form of calories only. . . . Alcohol taken to excess satisfies the immediate energy requirement, but the associate malnutrition and avitaminosis (vitamin deficiency) are manifested by fatty degeneration of the functioning organs of the body."

Dr. Butler adds that those who criticize or admonish the alcoholic probably cannot control their own diet, which keeps them overweight, or discontinue their smoking, which in some respects is an even more dangerous poison than alcohol.

Dr. Butler says that most authorities agree that, if an alcoholic will eat high-protein food every day, he will not suffer all the after-effects of alcoholism. An alcoholic patient who is put into a hospital and given an adequate diet with "intensive vitamin therapy" responds rapidly to this treatment. The problem is to get him to continue with the therapy after he is released. How do you do it? Get him to promise? Make a jailer and a dietician and a nurse out of his wife or mother or daughter?

Dr. Butler takes a simpler approach. He uses a precision diet consisting of a scientifically calculated liquid food that is pre-digested and placed directly into the patient's stomach. That's correct. Dr. Butler makes a small hole in the patient's stomach and fits a tube to it. This is plugged on the outside and the patient is given the liquid diet to take home if he wishes, or he can use it for only some meals, after he has once again established nutritious eating habits. If he has difficulty with the feeding, members of his family can help.

Dr. Butler described the treatment of a patient who had been a hopeless alcoholic for at least six years. He had not worked for three years and was admitted to the hospital in a state of acute delirium tremens with an accumulation of fluid in his lungs. He was taken to the operating room, a tube was inserted in his stomach. Within 48 hours he was walking around, needing nothing more than the prescribed feedings. After three months, he had gained 30 pounds and was working steadily.

Dr. Butler gives two other examples of this treatment and states that it is feasible for use in all other cases. The nutritional deficiency will be corrected and the nutritional complications of chronic alcoholism will be avoided. We agree completely with this idea and hope fervently that it may revolutionize alcoholic treatment in the United States.

You will note that Dr. Butler said alcohol is in the form of calories only. Hence, it is possible to subsist for a time on nothing but alcohol. The longer this goes on, of course, the more badly nourished one will be. What other substance is only empty calories? Sugar, of course. And it is possible to exist mainly on sugar for some time before multiple deficiencies begin to appear.

CHAPTER 4

More Nutritional Help for the Alcoholic

IN ITS RELATION to some other diseases, it seems likely that alcoholism and the other disorders all spring from a basic nutritional cause. A study of 841 tuberculosis patients in a veterans hospital showed that nearly half of them were alcoholics. A majority of the patients with hemorrhaging stomach and esophagus wounds were alcoholics. Of a group of patients with cancer of the pancreas, 75 per cent were alcoholics.

A survey of 922 employees of a large industrial firm who were known or suspected to be problem drinkers showed that they had a higher incidence of high blood pressure, cirrhosis of the liver, stomach ulcer, asthma, diabetes, gout, neuritis, cerebrovascular disease (which leads to strokes) and heart disease. Certainly, as we begin to relate all these conditions to inadequate nutritional support, it becomes evident that alcoholism is somehow tied in with the nutritional deficiency picture.

"A slow fire which tortures and eventually destroys its victims" is what Dr. Roger J. Williams called alcoholism in an address before the International Institute on Prevention and Treatment of Alcoholism in 1966. Throughout his address, Dr. Williams pleaded for more attention to the prevention of alcoholism, rather than trying to patch up the pieces that are left. What we must do, he said, is to "seek out all the potential causes and eliminate them as far as possible, without arguing inordinately about their relative importance."

Personality disorders and insecurity arising from early childhood events may be causes of alcoholism, he said, plus unwholesome attitudes toward drinking, lack of proper recreation and employment facilities. But equally important are glandular imbalance and poor nutrition.

"It is my opinion," he continued, "based upon about 20 years of study of the disease alcoholism, much of it intensive study, that nutrition has a great deal to do with alcoholism and that education in this area holds great promise for the prevention of the disease."

Why does it take several years at least, usually more, for the drinker to become an alcoholic? Dr. Williams points out that, as his intake of the drug increases, the alcoholic is not just becoming more and more poisoned by alcohol, but also less and less able to deal with life's daily problems because he is so poorly nourished.

Anyone who takes a considerable portion of his

calories as alcohol must eliminate from his diet an equal number of calories contained in good, wholesome, nutritious food. In Sweden, for example, it is estimated that the average alcohol consumption is 1,500 calories daily. Since the average total consumption of calories is 3,000, this means that half of the average Swede's calories come from alcohol, totally unaccompanied by anything nutritious at all.

Said Dr. Williams: "No one can claim to be eating wisely who regularly consumes quantities of 'naked' calories, either in the form of sugar or alcohol."

And if children were taught early the value of good nutrition and how to obtain it, he said, as well as the dangers of poor nutrition, we would have a sound basis for preventing alcoholism. He thinks that poor nutrition in childhood may be the chief factor that lays the groundwork for addiction to alcohol later in life.

At the same time Dr. Williams reviewed some of the animal experiments which we mentioned briefly in another chapter. Giving the animal a good diet with plenty of all the essential nutrients, he explained, reduces alcohol consumption to a low level. "This observation has been confirmed hundreds of times in many laboratories, so there is no question about it," Dr. Williams said.

Glutamine is one substance which Dr. Williams has found to be effective in alleviating alcoholism. That is, it can stop the desire to drink. It has been prescribed for patients who did not know they were getting it, did not know that they were being treated in any way. The craving for alcohol ceased. Other amino acids (or forms of protein) may be equally important, along with vitamins and minerals. Dr. Williams gives sources for glutamine in his books.

"I know of hundreds of alcoholics (and others who have not quite reached the compulsive stage) who have a substantial basis for thinking that they have been greatly benefited by the application of good nutrition to their problems," Dr. Williams said. "Physicians who care for alcoholics increasingly think of the importance of nutrition. Some reported effects of improved nutrition on alcoholics have been little short of miraculous. Why, then, is there varying success in the treatment of patients? Why do some patients respond and others do not?

"We speak loosely when we ascribe the diversity among alcoholics to their differing personalities," Dr. Williams said. "What is not commonly appreciated is that each one of us has a highly distinctive 'metabolic personality'—an internal biochemistry— of his own.

"While all of us make use of the very same amino acids, vitamins and minerals, the details of how we use them and the effectiveness with which we use individual nutrients varies endlessly in individual members of the human family," Dr. Williams continued. "In the matter of gastric digestive juices alone, one survey showed that, of 5,000 healthy individuals, the content of one digestive enzyme (pepsin) varies from zero to 4,300 units."

The same wide variability is characteristic of other parts of the body: blood, the shape and size of organs, glands, and so forth. "While in general we all need the same nutritional elements, amino acids, vitamins and minerals, the quantities of each that we need is highly distinctive for each of us," Dr. Williams noted.

"Recent experiments in our laboratory have shown this to be true of individual experimental animals, even when they are more closely related genetically than most human populations are. When 60 weaning rats were all fed a particular deficient diet, some died of malnutrition within a week, while others thrived in relatively good condition for nearly five months," Dr. Williams said. "Experiments of this type have been done repeatedly with both rats and mice, and the unequivocal conclusion is that, among these animals, the individual variation in nutritional needs is exceedingly high. There is not the slightest suggestion of a reason why these findings are not applicable in even a more striking way to human beings.

"There are many reasons why young people should be taught the dangers of malnutrition, even if there were no threat of alcoholism," the University of Texas scientist said. "The idea that all people are well nourished unless they can be proved to have a well recognized overt deficiency disease—such as beriberi or scurvy—is completely untenable and is based upon lack of appreciation of the fundamentals of nutritional biochemistry.

"Deficiencies can be severe," he said, "in which case overt disease develops, but they can also be relatively mild, in which case the deficiencies may go unrecognized. No one knows how many of the so-called metabolic diseases are aggravated and complicated by unobtrusive nutritional deficiencies related to the particular needs of the individuals concerned. . . . Children who are fed good diets eat less candy than children who get poor diets. Good diets promote good control mechanisms."

In an address before the Conference on Aging, sponsored by the Huxley Institute for Biosocial Research in 1972, Dr. Williams had this to say: "A most important part of the environment of an aging person is the food that he or she eats. This provides an internal environment for the cells and tissues. This environment is never perfectly adjusted. That it is poorly adjusted is due in part to the fact that our staple foods are often trashy and provide in a scanty fashion the nutritional essentials, which make possible the adequate maintenance and repair of body cells and tissues."

Continuing a theme that Dr. Williams has previously stressed, he said that, "There are two energy-yielding chemicals commonly consumed for which self-selection often fails to work advantageously. One is sugar. The other is alcohol. Children who are raised on soft drinks and given a choice will choose more of the same in preference to nourishing food. Adults who commonly consume alcoholic beverages regularly and copiously for long periods of time not infrequently reach the point where they lose interest in nourishing food and have, on the contrary, a prevailing interest in consuming alcoholic beverages.

"In each case," he stated, "the appetite-controlling

49

mechanism in the brain goes awry. In children, excess sugar consumption leads to general malnutrition. In adults, consuming too much alcohol can lead not only to general malnutrition, but also to severe damage of the brain. Brains of alcoholics are so badly damaged that their cadavers are unfit for brain dissection by medical students.

"Alcoholism is a terrible health hazard and elderly people are highly susceptible, particularly if they have had extended drinking experience," Dr. Williams said.

At the same Conference, Dr. George Christakis, a prominent nutrition specialist of Mt. Sinai School of Medicine in New York, told of a study in which four out of five subjects aged 50 to 70 required more total protein than younger men, particularly the two amino acids, lysine and methionine. He also commented on a survey of 3,000 elderly people which indicated a number of individuals with low levels of iron, vitamin A, vitamin C and vitamin B2.

In Texas and South Carolina, 3.2 per cent of all the elderly people surveyed were deficient in vitamin C, 8 per cent were deficient in vitamin B2 (riboflavin). He added significantly, "This does not include those individuals who may be receiving less than adequate nutritional care in nursing homes."

In a 14-year study of aging persons in California, 45 per cent of the women were found to be getting less than two-thirds of the recommended dietary allowance of calcium. Potassium, thiamine and other B vitamins are similarly lacking in many diets. And even though elderly people may be getting enough of all these elements at their meals, many conditions may prevent them from absorbing them: poor teeth or dentures, lack of digestive juices, diseases of the digestive tract and other diseases, as well as mental depression.

It is impossible, said Dr. Christakis, to buy nutritionally adequate meals on the welfare benefits received by many elderly people. For many reasons —like lack of mobility—it is difficult for older people to shop frequently for food. There is difficulty in storing food many times, lack of refrigeration, etc. Eating alone is depressing. Alcohol contributes calories in a pleasant, easy-to-prepare mixture. Dr. Christakis goes on to list the many complications that alcoholism may create for the elderly, because their aging condition makes them less able to withstand such onslaughts.

"At any rate, the thing to do is to eat adequate protein, obviously, and have all of the substrates, all of the micronutrients you need (he means vitamins and minerals), so when your body needs this turnover replacement, it can do it quite efficiently," Dr. Christakis said.

Dr. Abram Hoffer, also at the same Conference, told the story of the Canadian veterans of a World War II prison camp who came back to Canada in terrible shape. They had all the symptoms of mental illness. They complained constantly. They were depressed, fatigued, arthritic, neurotic. One friend of Dr. Hoffer's was in such a bad way that, by the age of 60, it took the combined efforts of him and his wife for one hour to get him out of bed every morning.

When Dr. Hoffer was working with niacin—or vitamin B3—which he gives in massive doses to mentally ill patients, this veteran became interested and began to take the vitamin himself, in massive doses. "Within two weeks this man had recovered and since that time he has remained well, with the exception of a period of two years later, when he went climbing the Rocky Mountains and forgot to take his vitamins with him," said Dr. Hoffer.

"So here we have one case which does not prove anything but does establish facts about a man who was brought back to health by the simple expedient of taking three grams a day of nicotinic acid (a form of niacin) . . . even though he had not expected any good to come out of it," Dr. Hoffer said.

Some of the other veterans began to take massive doses of the vitamin later, and, in spite of the terrible health handicaps they started with, they are now "as far as we can tell—normal," Dr. Hoffer said.

He added: "I think that senility is, in fact, merely a prolonged chronic form of malnutrition."

This is Dr. Hoffer's prescription for a diet and way of life that will "stave off senility:"

1. A good diet—plenty of high-quality protein, a proper balance of fats, *a marked reduction in sugars.*

2. Supplements.

a. Nicotinamide (a form of vitamin B3).

b. Nicotinic acid which lowers cholesterol, prevents "sludging" of the blood and helps to maintain the circulation.

c. Vitamin C. Dr. Hoffer gives this to his patients in very large amounts.

He told of giving as much as 90 grams a day to patients. "We have never yet seen any toxicity. If any person here doubts this, I will challenge you to a duel and will match you. You eat a spoonful of salt and I will eat a spoonful of ascorbic acid (vitamin C) and see who stops eating first." Dr. Hoffer, who, incidentally, is a psychiatrist in Saskatoon, Saskatchewan, Canada, and President of the Huxley Institute for Biosocial Research, takes four grams of vitamin C daily.

d. Pantothenic acid. This is the B vitamin discovered by Dr. Roger J. Williams.

e. Alpha tocopherol, vitamin E.

3. Dr. Hoffer mentioned many other factors in ill health: smoking, radioactive pollution, toxic metals which pollute air and water, and so on.

Later in the conference, Irwin Stone spoke of his work with vitamin C. He believes that it should not be called a vitamin. It is, instead, a substance essential for the liver. Be that as it may, humans do not manufacture their own vitamin C—as most animals and birds do—because of a mutation which occurred some 60 million years ago. He believes— and more and more scientists are coming around to his viewpoint—that research should be done giving, over long periods of time, enough of this substance to make up for what our livers would manufacture if we had not suffered the mutation so many years ago.

Someone inquired at the conference about the

possibility of such massive doses of vitamin C causing kidney stones. Dr. Hoffer said, "I have gone over the (medical) literature very carefully and so has Dr. Stone, he more carefully. So far, there is not a single report in the medical literature where this has been established. In fact, many physicians have recommended that ascorbic acid be used to dissolve kidney stones."

Dr. Williams had a final word on alcoholism.

"In my rather long clinical psychiatric experience, I have come to the conclusion, from which I would find it very hard to have my mind changed, that there is a qualitative difference between alcoholism occurring in people before the age of 35 and alcoholism occurring in the old-age category, whatever we call old age, let us say beyond 55 or 60.

"This is because, in most instances where I have treated what looked like real alcoholism in an older person it was much more readily reversible and even curable in the sense that the person could go back to social drinking, which is almost impossible with the young alcoholic.

"The reason, I think," Dr. Williams said, "is that so often alcoholism in an older person is based on depression. He is depressed and uses alcohol as his tranquilizer, whereas with younger people, depression follows alcoholism. It is a product of alcoholism."

In his recent book, *Nutrition Against Disease* (see Bibliography), Dr. Williams devotes a chapter to the subject of alcoholism.

New Hope for Incurable Diseases, by E. Cheraskin, M.D., D.M.D., and W. M. Ringsdorf, D.M.D., M.S. (see Bibliography), also contains an excellent chapter on alcoholism, including the diet for preventing low blood sugar, the use of megadoses of vitamins for treating alcoholism, and many more helpful suggestions and references. For information on Irwin Stone's book on vitamin C, also see the Bibliography.

Dr. Leevy tells us (*American Journal of Clinical Nutrition*, April 1965) that deficiency in vitamins often occurs in alcoholics in the complete absence of any symptoms of deficiency. Folic acid and pyridoxine, both B vitamins, are the two nutrients most often missing, he said. Studying the livers of alcoholics who were deficient in riboflavin, folic acid, pantothenic acid and pyridoxine (all B vitamins), he found that the changes wrought in the liver by these deficiencies could be reversed by giving the vitamins. Thiamine, another B vitamin, also improves the alcoholic's condition.

In *Biochemical Factors in Alcoholism*, published by Pergamon Press, Dr. Leevy tells us that both alcohol and dietary deficiency contribute to the fatty liver, the cirrhosis and other extremely serious disorders which plague the alcoholic. High protein intake and plenty of other essential nutrients can do much to rehabilitate the health of the alcoholic.

A recovery rate of 71 per cent has been achieved in a 2-year study of 507 alcoholics on massive doses of vitamin B3, according to Dr. Russell F. Smith, alcoholism expert of Brighton Hospital, Detroit,

Michigan. At the end of the test, 474 of the 507 patients were carefully studied. Of these, the 138 patients who were originally in "excellent" shape after a year of treatment were found to have suffered no relapses and to be in good emotional health. They had received no treatment but the vitamin. In a group called "good" at the end of the first year, 233 were continually sober and were moved up into the "excellent" category. "Nearly all these recoveries are today being maintained in Alcoholics Anonymous," according to an article in the American Schizophrenia Foundation publication. The Foundation is affiliated with The Huxley Institute for Biosocial Research.

Some of the benefits of the B3, or niacin, treatment are: marked ability of the vitamin to reduce the mood swings and insomnia common in alcoholics. It reduces or changes alcohol's effect on the individual. It reduces alcohol tolerance and the severity of withdrawal symptoms. It also stabilizes behavior in such a way that traditional treatments function more efficiently. Said Dr. Smith, while vitamin B3 itself is not a cure for alcoholism, "we are convinced that it is an important adjunct to traditional treatment of three out of four alcoholics."

In order to test the results of alcohol on B vitamins in the body, laboratory animals on their highly nutritious diet were given alcohol to drink and their urine was tested for B vitamins. Thiamine, pyridoxine and pantothenic acid were immediately excreted, as was a form of niacin. This abrupt increase in excretion of these important nutrients seems to show some kind of enzyme or metabolic disturbance, the researchers believe.

Some mice may be born alcoholics, said a headline in *New Scientist* for February 27, 1969. Three doctors from the University of Colorado describe experiments with two groups of mice on the same diet, some of whom continuously preferred alcohol to water, while others drank the water. The scientists found that the alcoholic mice had an excess of certain enzymes in their livers. Under ordinary circumstances laboratory mice do not have access to alcohol, so such a difference in make-up of liver enzymes would never have been discovered had this test not been done.

"One is forced to speculate, therefore, whether similar enzymatic patterns are of influence in those humans having a pathological penchant for alcohol," said *New Scientist*.

Another experiment involving laboratory mice on a deficient diet showed that niacin deficiency caused both male and female mice to turn to alcohol rather than water. When the diet was made nutritionally adequate—with plenty of vitamin B3 available—the consumption of alcohol dropped. This experiment was reported in the Quarterly *Journal of Studies of Alcoholism*, part A, 1969 (30)3, 592-7.

Rats which inhaled only polluted air during a 2-month experimental period chose to drink alcohol rather than water, a University of California researcher reported in June 1970. He does not know why and he has not tried his experiment with humans, because he would not expose them to such a high level of carbon monoxide. The rats were made to inhale air like that of automobile exhaust during constant bumper-to-bumper traffic. For the first three weeks, all the rats chose water rather than alcohol or sweetened beverages, But then the group exposed to the air pollution switched over to drinking alcohol. It's another indication that stress tends to addict us. And it is well to remember that cigarette smoke contains carbon monoxide, just as bumper-to-bumper traffic air does. Many humans find that smoking and drinking somehow go together.

"Not only does the chronic alcoholic not get enough vitamins, but in the process of burning alcohol in his system, he drains off what little amount of vitamins he may have acquired," says a note in *Science News Letter*, August 17, 1963. A University of California researcher tested alcoholics for vitamin deficiencies and found almost half of them had a vitamin B1 deficiency, while many had evidence of pyridoxine deficiency. Impaired nutrition undoubtedly underlies the actual nerve damage, which in the presence of alcohol brings on such hideous nerve disorders as the DT's.

A diet high in nutritional elements and low in calories is essential in the rehabilitation of alcoholics, said Dr. Gordon Bell of the Donwood Foundation for Alcoholics and Drug Addicts. He went on to say, in *The New York Times* for July 14, 1969, that the problem drinker gets up to 35 or 40 per cent of his calories from alcohol, causing an imbalance of proteins, vitamins and minerals. A frequent result is beriberi, the disease of vitamin B1 deficiency. The dietician at the Foundation plans meals high in protein and says that no patient should go longer than four hours without some kind of food. Alcoholics are notorious breakfast-skippers, she has found. And it is important to get at least one-quarter to one-third of one's calories at breakfast—every day.

The *British Medical Journal* for November 21, 1964 reported on three heavy drinkers who appeared to have some of the symptoms of beriberi. Breathlessness, swelling of the ankles and many kinds of heart irregularities were treated with massive doses of thiamine (vitamin B1) with good results.

Three Australian physicians reported in the July 10, 1971 issue of the *Lancet* on a 48-year-old alcoholic patient with brain deterioration due to long years of heavy drinking. Two weeks before he came to the hospital, he found he had difficulty in walking. He staggered and could not coordinate the movements of his legs. Other symptoms pointed to quite serious brain damage—the kind that heavy drinking eventually produces. He was given a richly nourishing diet and very high doses of vitamin B1. This was 200 milligrams by injection and 300 milligrams by mouth every day. The official recommendation for this vitamin for the average healthy adult, incidentally, is 1.4 milligrams daily.

So this alcoholic was getting more than 500 times the amount specified for a non-alcoholic. He was also given massive doses of vitamin B2 and vitamin B3. Within about three weeks he was able to leave the hospital and was given thiamine to take in massive doses. His symptoms improved and he was able to walk almost normally. Had he been able to stay on the wagon, the physicians are sure he could have recovered completely.

We generally think of cirrhosis of the liver as the classical disease of alcoholics. But many other conditions contribute to the ill-health of these unfortunates. *Archives of Internal Medicine* for October 1967 presented the case of a 36-year-old man suffering from heart failure and acute failure of the kidneys. He was found to be severely deficient in thiamine. So long had the deficiency been going on that his doctor thought that the man was suffering from beriberi. This patient had depended on alcohol for his calories to keep himself going; he had stopped eating nourishing food.

Since pure carbohydrate makes heavy demands on the body's store of vitamin B1, and, as we have mentioned, alcohol is pure carbohydrate, it is no wonder that this patient eventually degenerated into a beriberi patient. A massive dose of thiamine brought the kidneys back to normal, suggesting that the heart condition, brought on by the lack of thiamine, had caused the kidney condition.

In the *Journal of the American Medical Association* for May 1, 1967 there is a letter about the administration of large amounts of vitamins in injections for psychoses associated with alcoholism. Dr. N. T. Pollitt of London said that there appears to be some interference with the enzymes in the brain which enable the alcoholic to use sugar.

Saturation of the tissues with the B Complex and vitamin C restores normal function.

What does alcohol do to the heart? A November 1971 release from the National Institute of Health tells us that laboratory mice, given measured amounts of alcohol, developed weight gain, a build-up of fats in the myocardium (the muscular tissue of the heart), changes in heart cells and a loss of enzyme actions in the heart as a dircet result of alcohol consumption.

Furthermore, large doses of thiamine and multiple vitamin supplements often failed to reverse heart failure in alcoholic patients. In such cases, continued alcohol consumption results in further heart damage and eventually death. In such patients, the heart damage is probably due, in part at least, to alcohol's direct effect.

The heart, of course, is a muscle. A February 1972 release from NIH reports on experiments with human volunteers in which it was found that alcohol (42 per cent of the total calories) produced excessive amounts of a certain muscle enzyme and changes in skeletal muscles among the volunteers. All were supposedly eating a well-balanced diet. The volunteers were all occasional, moderate drinkers, not alcoholics.

Such an experiment leads one to believe that, if one is going to drink at all, even small, occasional drinks, there is an absolute necessity of including in one's diet an abundance of all those food elements that protect the health of muscles—and there are many.

Alcoholism is probably a contributing factor in hardening of the arteries, according to a team of Italian physicians. A psychiatric hospital in Rome admits about 6,000 patients yearly, of whom about 20 per cent are "pure" alcoholics—that is, they have not combined alcohol with drugs. When the doctors carefully studied 150 of these patients, they found evidence of hardening of the arteries in 81 per cent. Complicating the picture was the fact that most of them were also heavy smokers. In a series of tests, all 150 showed short-term memories, deficiencies in learning ability and loss of ability to adjust to new situations.

The Journal of the Dietetic Association of Australia discussed the nutritional aspects of alcoholism in the September 1967 issue. These are the ways in which alcoholism can lead to nutritional deficiency: There may be damage to the mouth, salivary glands, pancreas, liver, lining of the digestive tract. There may be "abnormal demands" for the B Complex and magnesium. The appetite may be depressed, resulting in deficiencies in iron, vitamins and proteins. Studying what the patients in their clinic ate, researchers found that most of them ate no breakfast, lunched on sandwiches or pies, usually had meat for dinner, but no vegetables or fruit. This is a diet that is bound to produce nutritional deficiencies.

In March 1966, four Toronto researchers reported that deficient diet, as well as heavy drinking has an effect on cirrhosis of the liver. The scientists said

that their studies showed that "most disadvantage-
ous effects of alcohol manifest themselves most dramatically when diets are low in protein and high in
sugar and starch. . . . Diets high in proteins of good
quality which contain only moderate amounts of
sugars and fats prevent almost completely the liver
alterations classically associated with excessive and
chronic consumption of alcohol." Food eaten by alcoholics should be extra high in vitamins and protein
content to offset the lack of vitamins and protein
in alcohol.

E. Rubin of Mt. Sinai Hospital in New York reported in *Gastronenterology*, for November 1972,
that alcohol produces striking changes in the lining
of the small intestines. They are similar to changes
produced in cells of the liver. The liver, of course,
is well known as the organ most frequently damaged
by alcoholism.

Research at Harvard University indicates that alcohol has perhaps as deleterious an effect on the
intestines as on the liver. Testing rats which were
given the same amount of alcohol a social drinker
might consume, Dr. Kurt Isselbacher found that the
increased fatty substances in the blood of the drinker
are related to the manufacture of fat in the intestines
as much as to liver fat. This was reported in the
January 14, 1972 issue of *Medical World News*.

And chronic alcoholism may result in severe depression of bone marrow, according to two Washington, D. C. physicians. This might explain the alcoholic's susceptibility to infection. The white blood

cells, whose job is to protect against infection, are manufactured in the bone marrow. When infection comes along the bone marrow is unable to produce an increase in these essential white blood cells, and the infection, unchecked, is likely to overwhelm the drinker.

"The association of alcoholism and pellagra is commonly seen in the Witwatersand area of South Africa," stated a letter to the editor of the *Lancet*, July 29, 1972. Pellagra, as you remember, is the vitamin B3 (niacin) deficiency disease. He goes on to speculate on what metabolic pathways might be involved with vitamins and amino acids which may bring on alcoholic symptoms, such as sleep disturbances, delirium, hallucinations and diarrhea.

Magnesium, an essential mineral, has been found to be lacking in chronic alcoholics. Giving the mineral as part of treatment of alcoholism resulted in improvement in the patient's appetite and mental attitude. This was reported in a German medical journal in 1968.

According to *Medical World News*, October 13, 1972, a Swedish researcher also believes that lack of magnesium may be responsible for the brain damage that occurs in alcoholism. Dr. Gustave Standig-Lindberg says that, even when DT's are present, there is no alcoholic damage to the brain tissues, if the alcoholic is getting enough magnesium. If not, brain damage results. It can be reversed in its early stages by "aggressive" magnesium therapy. Getting too little magnesium results in destruction of the capillaries—the tiniest of all the blood vessels. When capillaries in the nervous system are damaged, the brain is affected. For the record, the foods highest in magnesium are chiefly nuts, seeds, unprocessed, wholegrain cereals of all kinds.

In a letter to the editor of *Medical Tribune*, January 19, 1972, Dr. L. F. Rutter of England said, in part: "It is well recognized by those concerned with alcoholics that a considerable proportion show schizoid symptoms: aberrations of the perceptive senses such as touch, sight and hearing.

"Typical descriptions of symptoms are 'I feel as if I'm walking on cotton wool,' or 'Things sometimes appear to me as if I'm looking through the wrong end of a telescope,' also 'hearing voices or funny sounds' and 'I thought I smelt peculiar.' Fear of impending insanity is also given by some as a reason for continued drinking . . . 'I blot out the horrid thoughts.'"

Dr. Rutter went on to point out that, in a test group of abstinent and long-recovered alcoholics, he found that they were unable to deal with a certain amino acid which converts into vitamin B3 in the body. So, he said, it is possible that such alcoholics suffer from a gross deficiency in niacin. Since alcoholics and schizophrenics seem to have at least this in common, schizophrenics should be expected to benefit from vitamin B3 treatment.

The fatty substances which build up in blood and liver after even a moderate amount of drinking may threaten social drinkers as well as alcoholics, according to Dr. Emanuel Rubin and Charles S. Lieber of Mt. Sinai School of Medicine. Their volunteers drank for about a week "socially," not to excess. The drinks produced a 5- to 13-fold increase in fatty substances in the liver—this in spite of a high-protein diet and vitamin supplementation. Three Canadian physicians have found they can prevent the build-up of fat with plenty of vitamins and related substances which tend to offset fatty accumulations. And a 1967 report from Australia indicates that levels of fatty substances in the blood rise rapidly "to extreme levels" when one is drinking alcohol and tend to fall when the alcohol is withdrawn. Uric acid also appears in excess with heavy drinking.

The Journal of Nutrition reported in July 1969 that drinking alcohol before or during a high-fat meal increases the usual amounts of fats in the blood. An enzyme in the intestines is inactivated by alcohol and a high-protein meal stays much too long in the stomach, when it is accompanied by several drinks.

Drinking one ounce of alcohol every day could have the same effect on a person's chromosomes as total body exposure to one roentgen a week of ionizing radiation, said two University of Georgia researchers. Alcohol breaks up chromosomes—those tiny parts of cells which carry inherited information from one generation to the next. If they are disordered, defective children are likely to result. Coffee produced somewhat the same effects in these tests. True, said the experimenters, both alcohol and coffee are metabolized rapidly by the body, which would lessen the deleterious effects somewhat. But, even so, any young person (of child-bearing age) takes a chance of having deficient children if he or she drinks excessively either alcohol or coffee.

Another symptom which seems to link alcoholism with genetic inheritance is the finding that a disproportionately large number of alcoholic men are color blind. Color blindness is an inherited defect. Now it appears it may be linked with a susceptibility to alcoholism.

The American Journal of Psychiatry for January 1966 reported that 40 per cent of all drivers responsible for fatal motor accidents were alcoholics and 10 per cent were pre-alcoholic. Many of the alcoholic drivers had a long history of serious psychopathology which may have contributed to their accident susceptibility. More than 50 per cent of them were paranoid (imagining that people around them were enemies), others were violent, depressed or suicidal.

Physicians at the Caroline Institute in Stockholm are sure that a dose of vitamins *before* drinking will help the drinker to feel less drunk. They injected a number of volunteers with B vitamins, another group with a dummy solution. All of them drank a given amount of alcohol, but those who had received the B vitamins came out better in tests than the others.

Scientists have known for many years that a diet in which there are large amounts of uncooked egg white may bring about a deficiency in biotin, a B vitamin. The reason is a protein—called avidin—which exists in raw egg whites. This substance latches onto the biotin and makes it unavailable to the body. The individual who eats large amounts of raw eggs will probably become deficient in this vitamin. Cooking inactivates the avidin.

Such a case was seen by physicians at the Medical College of Birmingham, Alabama and reported in the *American Journal of Clinical Nutrition* for February 1968. A 62-year-old woman came to the hospital with alarming symptoms. She had no appetite, her mouth and lips were sore, she had a scaly dermatitis. Further, she suffered from nausea and vomiting, mental depression, pallor, muscle pains and pains around her heart. She also had tingling and pricking sensations in her hands and feet. The doctors did the usual tests and found that she had anemia, abnormal heart action, extremely high cholesterol levels and certain liver symptoms. They asked her what she had been eating to get into this state. Here is what she said.

She had suffered from cirrhosis, a kind of liver disorder probably brought on by rather heavy drinking earlier in life. Her doctor wanted her to get lots of excellent protein, so he told her to eat, every day, six raw eggs and two quarts of milk, in addition to her regular food. She did this for 18 months. After a few weeks on this diet, she lost her appetite, but, since she wanted to obey her doctor's orders, she went on with the raw eggs and milk. She also took a vitamin capsule which the doctor had prescribed for her. However, it contained no biotin. She also took several brewer's yeast tablets.

"Thus," noted the authors of the article, "the stage was set for development of biotin deficiency." Her symptoms developed rapidly and she was in serious condition when she came to the Alabama hospital. After they had taken her history, the doctors immediately tested her for biotin and found that she was deficient in this B vitamin. They gave her injections of biotin and, within three days, all her symptoms began to disappear.

When she was discharged, cured, she was told not to eat uncooked eggs and was placed on a high-protein diet. Several months later she had great emotional stress when her husband died, and she stopped eating the prescribed diet, developed a fever and cough and had trouble sleeping. When she came back to the hospital, the doctors gave her injections of biotin again and her symptoms disappeared.

Although eggs are an excellent food and should be eaten daily, don't eat raw eggs in abundance. Obviously, six raw eggs per day is far more than anyone with any nutritional background would recommend. But don't neglect eggs, either alone or in your cooking. There is still not enough convincing evidence that the cholesterol in eggs is harmful, especially since eggs also contain lecithin, an emulsifier, which probably helps to break up the cholesterol so that it does not clog the arteries.

And when you are selecting a food supplement, try to get one which contains all 11 vitamins of the B Complex, even the obscure ones like biotin. The official booklet, *Recommended Dietary Allowances*, says this about biotin: "Daily needs are provided by diets containing 150 to 300 micrograms of biotin.

This amount is provided by the average American diet." Obviously, this was not the case with the patient we have just discussed. It may not also be true for those of us who have a higher than normal need for biotin, especially if we are under stress. And alcoholism is certainly one form of stress.

A Michigan company is developing a pill which they believe will sober-up anyone who has had too much liquor. It consists of dried food yeast with vitamin B1, vitamin B2 and vitamin B3. They have tested this product on hundreds of people and declare that it works, that people who have taken inordinate amounts of liquor and are drunk, according to all criteria, can be sober within a half hour or so after they have taken the pills. They are presently offering the pills for sale.

CHAPTER 5

The Tragedy of Teen-Age Drunks

"EVERY PARENT OF adolescent children knows that in recent years increasing numbers of teen-agers have been experimenting with dangerous drugs— LSD, speed, barbiturates, even heroin," reports the March 5, 1973 issue of *Newsweek*.

"Perhaps the most frightening aspect of this trend is that in well-to-do suburban communities and inner-city ghettos alike the age of the youthful drug experimenters has been steadily dropping; there have even been cases of heroin addiction among elementary school children.

"Now, however," *Newsweek* continued, "the trend seems to be away from these drugs. From nearly every quarter of the nation, school authorities and teen-agers themselves report that the latest fad in juvenile drug abuse is . . . alcohol."

The article stated that, " 'Clearly, one reason for the proliferation of young drinkers is widespread tolerance by their parents, most of whom are drinkers themselves. Parents who hassled their kids about other drugs are willing to look the other way on alcohol,' stated Norm Southerby of the Los Angeles County Alcohol Safety Action Program."

Southerby told· about the parents of a 19-year-old girl who had experienced such anguish because she was a heavy user of pot and pills. They were "deeply relieved" when she began drinking, even though "she'd get so drunk that she would be throwing up in the morning." He stated that one teen-ager out of every 20 in Southern California "has a drinking problem," *Newsweek* noted. Los Angeles County is trying to educate children against the problems of drinking with a new film, "99 Bottles of Beer."

"In a recent study of youthful drinking habits in the upper-middle-class Boston suburb of Brookline, 36 per cent of the 8th-grade pupils reported having been drunk on wine or beer—and so did 14 per cent of the 6th-grade class," the magazine reported.

There were other cases of older teen-agers "pushing booze" to younger students. And at Levittown Memorial High School on Long Island, N. Y., a 17-year-old member of the football and lacrosse teams "reports that on Saturday evenings in good weather, about a hundred 15- to 17-year-olds regularly congregate in the bleachers of the playing field to consume a six-pack of beer apiece. After these weekend binges, says Frank Trezza, the school's director of student organizations, the playing area may be littered with as many as 250 empty beer cans, fifteen wine bottles and several whisky bottles," *Newsweek* continued. Another student reported that "alcohol is just as much fun as grass, and a lot easier to obtain."

In San Francisco, a top student and member of the swimming team at Woodrow Wilson High School popped some pills, pushed them down with several drinks—and was found dead the next morning, the magazine said.

Continued *Newsweek*: " 'Teen-agers have always used alcohol,' points out Milton Wolk of the alcoholism division of the Massachusetts Department of Public Health, 'and they always will. And because teen-age use is patterned after adult use, there's no way kids are going to stop drinking until adults do.' "

"College students appear to be turning off hard drugs and turning into the narcotic of their elders—alcohol," said the *New York Daily News*, March 12, 1973. A City College student is quoted as saying that "You can go into any lounge here after the Thursday club break, and it looks like one great New Year's Eve party . . . there are drunks all over the place."

Students, of course, have not stopped using drugs entirely; marijuana is often smoked openly in classrooms and dorms. There are several reasons why college students are turning away from the hard stuff: it's expensive, they now realize that it can harm their health, and they've been through that scene in high school.

Said the *Daily News*: "Liquor stores near college campuses are showing marked increases in sales this year—especially in cheap fruit wines." Students at Hunter College and Columbia University said that the "in" meeting places are now bars.

However, a growing problem with the young pill-poppers is a family of drugs called methaqualones, which some experts believe are as great a problem as heroin. This was the theme of NBC's magazine series, "First Tuesday," which was broadcast March 6, 1973.

Discussing the program in the March 1, 1973 issue of the *New York Post*, Bob Williams said: "Producer Bob Rogers, who prepared the report, says some experts regard the methaqualones—sedative hypnotic narcotics which were designed to replace barbiturates as sleeping pills—as the hottest drug in America today and the biggest drug problem right now."

In the just-named *Daily News* article, a Brooklyn College student is quoted as saying that the methaqualones are "definitely up-and-comers. They're fun —everything feels so good and you just love everyone."

Continued Bob Williams: "Youngsters got into the drugs (methaqualones) under the brand names of Sopor and Quaalude, among others, according to Rogers, because they were supposed to be 'safe' and non-habit forming, but reports are now coming in of fatal overdoses.

"Young people are taking Sopor everywhere, at Sopor parties, dances, and rock concerts, and an increasing number are turning up in hospital emergency rooms. . . . The biggest problem is that this stuff is addictive but most kids don't know that and, therefore, are getting themselves hooked on what is a 'safe' drug.

"The irony, according to Rogers, is that the methaqualones are not on the federal government's list of controlled drugs. Nobody knows how many methaqualones the drug companies are putting out. . . . One thing we do know is that sales of methaqualones are rising . . . and so are thefts of the drug from warehouses and doctors' offices."

Because of the increasing problem with methaqualone, the New York State Health Department announced that, on April 1, 1973, this drug would be included in the new Controlled Substances Law, along with some other commonly abused prescription drugs—methadone, morphine, amphetamines, to name three.

"Several physicians involved in drug treatment programs have said that methaqualone can be addictive and that the addiction is tougher to kick than a heroin habit," said the *New York Post*, March 27, 1973. "Overdoses are known to have caused delirium, coma, internal bleeding and death."

Under the new procedure, physicians can only prescribe methaqualone on a special registered form, a copy of which must be sent to the Health Department, along with the patient's and doctor's names and addresses. Prescriptions are only in effect for 30 days, at which time they can only be refilled by another visit to the doctor.

"This procedure should help restrict the flow of methaqualone to the illegal market," stated Dr.

Hollis S. Ingraham, New York State Health Commissioner.

A recent study, reported at an American Medical Association drug conference by Dr. George R. Gay, stated that the heroin "epidemic" in the San Francisco Bay area—and perhaps the nation—is coming to an end. New heroin addicts seen at the Haight-Ashbury Free Medical Clinic have declined sharply in 1971-72, compared to the peak years of 1969-70, said *American Medical News,* December 18, 1972. Said Dr. Richard S. Wilbur, Assistant Secretary of the Defense Department for Health and Environment, at the same conference: "Heroin abuse in the armed forces has been brought under control—although it is still a serious problem." Two years ago, it was totally out of hand, he said.

The October 2, 1972 issue of the *Chicago Tribune* carried Part II of a series, "Alcohol Found to Be Major Teen Problem." Written by Science Editor Ronald Kotulak, the article said that the following alarming statistics had been released by public health officials:

"1) Drinking is widespread among teen-agers. Many have had their first taste of an alcoholic beverage by the age of 13.

"2) A study of boys in seven junior and senior high schools in the Boston area disclosed that by the time they graduated nearly one of every 14 was a confirmed alcoholic.

"3) Alcoholic beverages are being used along with marijuana and other drugs because teen-agers have discovered that alcohol speeds the absorption of the drugs into their blood.

"4) During the last 10 years, arrests of girls 18 years and younger who were intoxicated by liquor have more than tripled and arrests of boys in the same age group have jumped about 2½ times, said Dr. Morris E. Chafetz, director of the National Institute of Alcohol Abuse."

Stated Phyllis K. Snyder, director of the Chicago Alcoholic Treatment Center: "We first noticed the increase in teen-age alcoholics about two years ago. Now we have a regular referral service for them to appropriate treatment centers. . . . They think it is romantic to drink wine and smoke pot by candlelight, but it is a tragic combination."

Expanding on the previous study of Boston-area schools, Dr. Harold W. Demone, Jr., a Harvard University psychiatrist and executive director of the United Community Services of Metropolitan Boston, said that his study of 3,500 boys in (the Boston schools) showed that by the time they reached 18 years of age, 85 per cent were either light, moderate, heavy, relief or pathological drinkers, the *Tribune* reported. In addition, by the age of 14, 1.3 per cent of the boys were pathological drinkers. The number of alcoholics among the boys steadily increases to 7 per cent by the time they are 18 and over.

"These boys," Dr. Demone said, "were they adults, would be described as problem drinkers or Alcoholics."

The *Tribune* further quoted Dr. Demone as saying that the hallmark of an excessive teen-age drinker is that he is unhappy, his home life is inadequate, he probably has parents who are problem drinkers, he engages in antisocial activities, and he does poorly in school.

Although these problems are obviously a contributing factor to teen-age drinking, we would suggest that a major reason for today's terrible toll in alcoholism—among adults as well as teen-agers—is because of bad dietary practices and the alarming national sugar consumption of the past 25 years. We are exploring this thesis in greater detail in other chapters. However, children brought up to swill soft drinks all day can, as young adults, turn to alcoholic drinks and get from them the same energy and the same lift. Just as alcohol keeps one going seemingly without the need for food, so soft drinks and other empty calorie foods like candy, processed cereals, potato chips, etc., can be made to substitute for real food. A recent survey by *Boy's Life* magazine showed that 8 per cent of its readers drink eight or more bottles of pop a day.

Meanwhile, eating habits become worse and worse, and the individual depends more and more on his calorie crutch to keep going, as we have noted in other chapters on alcoholism. Before he knows it, he's either a sugar addict or an alcoholic, unable to get along for any length of time without the boost of another soft drink, another candy bar, another highball.

"In May 1886," reports the *New York Post*, January 10, 1973, "a pharmacist in Atlanta, a certain Dr. John Pemberton, invented a tonic by combining the extracts of the cocaine-containing coca leaves and the African kola nut with carbonated water. His tonic, which he called Coca-Cola, was an instant success.

"In 1906," the *Post* continued, "the federal government ruled that 'coke' could no longer be added to Coca-Cola and other beverages, but some 500 tons of 'de-cocained' coca leaves are still imported to this country from South America for use in soft drinks." Earlier in the century numerous patent medicines were widely sold whose chief ingredient was cocaine. In a later chapter on low blood sugar, we will show what happens to the Qolla Indians in Peru. One of their vices is chewing the coca leaf.

Sigmund Freud, the father of modern orthodox psychiatry, was a user of cocaine. He saw the drug as a virtual panacea for many afflictions. He used it for his migraine headaches and "to help in his writing," according to the *Post*.

Science News for May 23, 1970 reported that many hyperactive children are known to be susceptible to other psychological disorders, especially alcoholism, in later life. A follow-up study of 50 hyperactive children showed that a high proportion of the parents of these children were alcoholics themselves. Twenty-four per cent of the fathers and 4 per cent of the mothers of hyperactive children were alcoholics and 18 per cent of the grandfathers of hyperactive children were probable or definite alcoholics. We have more to say about hyperactive, hyperkinetic, problem children in the section on mental illness.

One out of every 15 young persons will become an alcoholic unless there is a change in environment and attitude toward drinking, the chairman of the AMA committee on alcoholism said in 1965. "In about 10 per cent of the cases of alcoholism, we find the individual is alcoholic from the very first drink."

New Scientist for September 1972 tells us that British authorities are now concerned about drinking in the 15-18-year-old group who patronize discotheques. "Prolonged drinking, often coupled with an inadequate diet, can cause vitamin deficiency disease, and in some cases weakens the heart muscle . . . as well as skeletal muscle.

"It is well known that alcohol widens the cerebral ventricles in the brain as it creates dementia, and Noble has recently demonstrated that heavy alcohol consumption decreases brain protein synthesis. Various anemias are now known to be associated with alcohol. . . . Alcoholic pancreatitis, decreased immune response, decreased phagocytosis of white blood cells, peripheral neuritis, osteoporosis (softening of the bone structure), and endocrine effects have also become apparent and more easily studied," *New Scientist* stated.

Dr. Carroll M. Leevy of the New Jersey College of Medicine, Jersey City, believes that a nutritious diet is essential for recuperation of the alcoholic. And he must abstain. He has found deficiency of folic acid and vitamin B12, both B vitamins, in alcoholics.

Since human beings cannot be placed in laboratories, scientists must, of necessity, experiment with animals. Tests with rats at Loma Linda University showed that the previous nutritional state influences one's susceptibility to alcohol addiction. Dr. U. D. Register and his colleagues said that they are "tentatively concluding that the craving for alcohol may come from a chemical imbalance created by the inadequate diet." The diet referred to was called "The teen-age diet" by the scientists. It was high in sugar and other carbohydrates and low in vitamins and minerals.

They gave their laboratory rats doughnuts and coffee for breakfast; sweet rolls and coffee for coffee breaks at 10 a.m. and 3 p.m.; hot dogs and mustard, relish, soft drinks, apple pie and coffee for lunch; spaghetti and meatballs, white bread, green beans, chopped salad, chocolate cake and coffee for dinner; candy bar, cookies and coffee for pre-bedtime snack.

On this diet, 80 per cent of the rats chose to drink dilute alcohol rather than water and they soon became addicted to the alcohol. *They could not do without it.* The other 20 per cent steadfastly drank water until the water was sweetened with about as much sugar as one cocktail might contain. Then they switched to drinking alcohol. When half of the rats were put on a nourishing diet, they immediately began to drink from one-tenth to one-fifth less alcohol. The remaining rats, which continued on the "teen-age diet," continued to drink heavily.

Over a 16-week period, those rats which continued to eat the deficient diet were drinking what would be, for a human, a quart of whisky a day. Supplementing this diet with vitamins and minerals, the scientists found that the rats soon began to drink one-third less alcohol. The researchers speculate that there is something in diet, aside from vitamins and minerals, which influences how much alcohol is consumed. This research was presented at a meeting of the Federation of American Societies for Experimental Biology in April 1970.

How many youngsters do you know who are trying to subsist on the above "teen-age diet?"

CHAPTER 6

The Magnitude and Seriousness of the Drug Problem

"MELANIE R. WAS buried in a green Long Island cemetery yesterday, 7,500 miles from the primitive, dusty city where she died 12 days ago at the end of an unaccomplished search for 'nirvana,' as she once put it," reported *The New York Times*, November 17, 1972.

"Melanie—that is not her real name—19 years old, died after smoking 26 pipes of opium, leaving in the flophouse (in Kabul, Afghanistan) where she spent her last days her Bonwit Teller and Lord & Taylor charge-account cards, her student card from Emerson College in Boston, a letter from her distraught mother, a sleeping bag, and a carpet bag containing a few clothes and odds and ends."

Melanie, who unfortunately is typical of many college-age youngsters in the United States, presented her well-traveled passport in the U.S. Embassy in Kabul, said that she had just arrived from Teheran, would stay about two weeks, and then go on to India. After leaving the United States, she had traveled extensively in France, Israel, Turkey, Greece, Ethiopia and elsewhere.

"Those who had lived with her at the Green Hotel . . . with three or four beds in each room, said that they had not gotten to know her well between her arrival Oct. 29 and her death but that she had been stoned all the time," the *Times* reported.

". . . Melanie walked out into the night from the New Istalif (a hotel)—no one knows how and when—and collapsed on the sidewalk near the Green Hotel. She was found there early Sunday and died at 2 o'clock in the afternoon in the Hospital for Women."

Back in the States, her friends and teachers described Melanie as "a nice girl, a good girl, well-mannered . . . but shy and confused." Explained a friend, "and the more confused she got, the deeper she got into drugs."

In Israel, where she attended Tel Aviv University for a time, Melanie had apparently only smoked hashish. But when the school term ended she began spending time in Elath, on the Gulf of Agaba, "where a group of expatriates lived in little huts and had access to opium and other hard drugs." Later she began "tripping" with LSD and thinking about suicide.

Continued the *Times*, "In a country where thousands are starving to death for want of food or money (in Afghanistan), the young transients are ill-nourished, though they have money, traveler's checks or credit cards in their pockets, because opium and hashish cause them to neglect all else. Experts here attribute the frequent deaths among them more to general debilitation and lowered resistance to the manifold ailments of this undeveloped country than to overdoses of narcotics.

"Americans make up about a fifth of the transients, whose annual wave begins in May, peaks during the summer and falls off in November," the *Times* said. "Last year's total was 61,000 tourists in a country with one decent hotel. From here most of the young travelers continue across the Khyber Pass toward Katmandu, Nepal, the other main station of the hashish pilgrimage.

"Although most are noticeably unwashed and their clothes are shabby, they do not appear to be poor," the *Times* continued. "Americans who run out of money get more from home, according to embassy officials. In three years only two have had to be repatriated by the embassy for lack of funds.

"For the last week of her life, Melanie was one of the few hundred Americans and Western European transients in the flophouses in the Shar-i-Nau section of this disheveled mountain capital, where a bed costs 20 afghanis (25 cents) a night," the *Times* said.

On one of the walls of a hotel that Melanie patronized, this menu was posted: "Acid, $1 . . . Opium, 30 afghanis . . . heroin, 7 afghanis."

"The estimated number of heroin addicts in the United States has multiplied 12 times in the last 10 years, an official of the Justice Department's Office of National Narcotics Intelligence said yesterday," stated *The New York Times* on December 14, 1972.

"Dan McAuliffe told the annual convention of the National Association of Citizen Crime Commissions that there were an estimated 600,000 heroin addicts in the country today, as compared with 50,000 ten years ago.

"He said that while the rate of heroin addiction is far higher now, it is increasing at a slower rate," the *Times* reported.

More than 30,000 of New York City's estimated 150,000 heroin addicts now receive daily maintenance doses of methadone. Methadone is a "harmless" drug on which a heroin addict can somehow manage to get along without heroin, but, of course, he then becomes addicted to the methadone. And, inevitably, methadone is now circulating as an illicit drug, since those who possess it can slip a few pills to other addicts who can't get it from legal channels.

Methadone has some quite serious side effects. Although it blocks the effects of heroin and satisfies the addict's craving for heroin, the patient feels no special effects from methadone, so he is, generally speaking, much more able to get a job and sustain himself in the community without difficulty. However, most addicts on methadone complain of constipation, about half of them perspire profusely, some gain weight, others have nightmares, while still others suffer from sleep disturbances. Withdrawing from methadone is an even worse experience than withdrawing from heroin addiction. But, according to the *New York Post*, "in both cases the symptoms are no worse than a bad case of the flu."

One reason for the inability of Asians to understand our revulsion to the trade in heroin (which comes from poppies) is that they use the raw material from the poppies they grow for medicine. "Is it true," they were quoted as asking (*National Observer*, February 10, 1973) "that people boil it, turn it into powder, and stick it in their arms with a needle? Why do they do that? Everybody knows it's *ya fin*, medicine, that you take it for your stomach or to go to sleep at night?" An American commented, "We often think of the reaction an Idaho farmer would have if some foreigner came along and told him to stop growing potatoes, because people overseas were getting drunk on vodka, which is made out of potatoes."

Nearly half the high school students in the New York Public School system—the nation's largest— are drug users, and in the junior high grades, the figure is 20 per cent, according to the state commission of education. Further, 75 per cent of high school students now drink alcoholic beverages. Alcoholics Anonymous now counts a growing number of young people in its ranks. The average age of an A.A. member used to be 45; now it is 33.

Almost everybody agrees that marijuana, or pot, is much less harmful than other drugs, and that it is not addictive in the true sense of the word. A letter to Ann Landers from an unnamed high school teacher in an Oklahoma city said this about those students in her classes who habitually smoke pot: "Their reactions to almost everything become distorted. They become lethargic, passive and depressed. On Mondays especially they come to class stoned and fall asleep during study period. The most frightening part of all is that they cannot think straight. That teen-agers should take such a chance with their precious mental machinery horrifies me. . . . I love kids and I hate to see what marijuana is doing to them."

Although exact figures are not available, it is estimated that perhaps as many as 5,700 of America's 287,000 physicians may be drug addicts. Addiction among physicians has been described as "a major problem." They have easy access to all kinds of drugs and presumably plenty of confidence that they will not become addicted because they know how to avoid addiction—they think. But, according to one specialist, the ones who are most confident are the ones who "get hooked" the worst. Doctors who become addicts complain of being ill, tired and overworked. So why do they take drugs? Could it perhaps be a nutritional deficiency?

A 1969 study of all junior and senior high students in the nation's tenth largest public school system (almost 57,000 students) revealed that 28 per cent had experimented with illicit drugs, 8 per cent had used them more than 10 times, and 4 per cent had used them frequently. The most commonly reported drugs were alcohol, tobacco, glue (to sniff), marijuana, solvent inhalants and pep pills.

In England, heroin is a legal drug which doctors may prescribe for addicts. Consequently, there is no black market there and no need for addicts to become criminals to support a heroin habit involving large sums of money. Doctors register their heroin addict patients and give them minimum doses daily.

In the *Journal of the American Medical Association* for January 29, 1973, Dr. Edward Lewis, Jr. considered the prospect of a similar program for this country. Dr. Lewis said, after careful study of the British method, that he does not think it would work in the United States, mostly because we lack a National Health System under which a physician can devote full time to treatment of addicts if he wishes. The American physician finds that even a small number of addicts and/or alcoholics disrupts his practice and makes it nearly impossible to continue. Since we already have a methadone program, why switch over to heroin now when it appears that the British may be coming around gradually to emulating our own methadone procedures?

In 1960 the number of babies born to addicted mothers in New York City was one in each 164 deliveries. In the first half of 1972, it was one in every 40 deliveries. Babies born to mothers addicted to heroin or methadone must be treated with drugs when they have moderate or severe withdrawal symptoms.

"A special legislative committee reported that at least 550 children were born addicted to drugs in New York City in 1971, suffering from withdrawal symptoms because their mothers had been using heroin or methadone," said *The New York Times* on November 2, 1972.

"Peter J. Costigan, chairman of the Assembly

Committee on Child Abuse, said there might have been as many as 2,000 such births. The Suffolk Republican added that 'untreated, a newborn's addiction can be fatal.'

"Unfortunately, we have found only a haphazard response on the part of the responsible city agencies to this grave and increasing problem."

Continued the *Times:* "The committee's executive director, Douglas J. Besharov, said a study by the Nassau County Medical Center had reported that the death rate among untreated babies with withdrawal symptoms varies from 50 to 95 per cent."

How drugs taken during pregnancy may affect the fetus in the womb, at birth or later in life was explored by an international panel of experts in pediatrics, obstetrics, pharmacology and related fields on March 15-16, 1973 at Hotel Commodore, New York City. Called "Drugs and the Unborn Child," the symposium was sponsored by the National Foundation—March of Dimes and presented by Cornell University Medical College.

"The immediate effects of drugs pregnant women take may be observable, but the long-term potential in terms of birth defects is wholly unknown," stated Dr. Wallace W. McCrory, professor and chairman of pediatrics, Cornell Medical Center.

"We simply do not know the price our children may be paying for drugs which affect their first environment," Dr. McCrory said.

The symposium was not confined to hard drugs, but to such things as alcohol, pep pills, aspirin, reducing pills, tobacco, cough and cold remedies, tranquilizers, sedatives, antacids, etc., along with marijuana, "psychedelic" drugs and other narcotics.

"Many things contribute to differences in individual reactivity to drugs," stated a background paper for the meeting. "A major factor is genetic. There are by now at least 20 or so well-established genetic traits associated with abnormal reactions to one or more drugs; some traits are vulnerable to a whole array of widely used medications. New ones are being discovered at a steady pace.

"These are a part of polymorphic genetic heritage of man and are often classified with inborn errors of metabolism in which the 'error' causes disease only when the bearer of a trait is exposed to a particular drug. If the bearer is a fetus, the exposure to even a small amount of a drug may lead to his death, malformation, growth retardation or late onset type of functional deficit . . .

"But drugs and poisons, like Jekyll and Hyde, are two faces of the same entity. Drugs make adults sick and account for perhaps 10 per cent of hospital admissions (Johns Hopkins study). It will be surprising if the unborn child is more resistant to drugs than grown men and women. This commonplace deduction is perhaps enough to justify all the cautionary remarks of physicians, government, the communications media and The National Foundation."

Another form of sickness is the large number of child abuse cases turning up in major cities. During a visit to New York on April 24, 1973 Senator Walter Mondale (D., Minn.), whose Senate Subcommittee is sponsoring the proposed Child Abuse Prevention Act, visited facilities for the Roosevelt Child Abuse Committee. He held a 2½-year-old girl, admitted the week before, who had a large lump on her forehead, two badly bruised eyes and old scars on her legs, believed to be from cigarette burns. The Senator also saw colored slides of a 7-month-old child bitten by his father; the child had deep skin lesions and was suffering from a brain hemorrhage. Another case showed a child with marks from severe strapping, reported the *New York Post* on April 24, 1973.

"The parents of one out of every four abused children in New York should not be allowed to resume care of their children, the Senate's Children and Youth Subcommittee was told today. The figure is far higher than the national average," the *Post* stated.

Dr. Marianne Schwob, chairman of the Roosevelt Child Abuse Committee, is quoted as saying that, "In New York there is a higher incidence of psychotic families who are on drugs and cannot be relied on to take back their children. It is our experience that only 75 per cent of the city's abused children should be returned to their parents."

Barbara Blum, assistant administrator of special services for children in the Human Resources Administration, testified that, for the first two months of 1973, 2,500 children had been reported to the city's central registry as suspected child abuse cases, the *Post* continued. Mrs. Blum's department projected 15,000 reports for 1973, or 5,000 more than in 1972. Of the 1972 total, 1,400 cases were of children under one year old.

"We have a population of 130,000 under one year old in New York, which means we're getting 1 in 10 reported as suspected cases of child abuse," Mrs. Blum told the *Post*.

Disagreeing with an earlier figure we have quoted in this book, Mrs. Blum estimated that as many as 1,500 city children were born drug addicted annually and in the first days of life experienced the tremors of withdrawal.

Heroin pushers sell an estimated $6 billion worth of the stuff yearly and it seems impossible to control the flow of the drug from the Eastern countries— where it is mostly grown—to U. S. cities.

"Four sleek planes hauled the marijuana from deep inside Mexico to a pair of elegant villas in San Luis, just below the U.S. border," stated the March 26, 1973 issue of *Newsweek*. "There it was packed into bricks and stored in underground cellars hidden beneath giant haystacks. An elaborate distribution system was set up to shuffle the stuff into the U.S.

"But the big pot party never got off the ground," *Newsweek* continued. "A joint team of U.S. and Mexican agents raided the operation last month, arresting 117 people and seized a mind-blowing 24.5 tons of Mexican grass. It was the biggest such bust ever. And it pointed up the newest wrinkle in pot smuggling—a massive Mexican airlift that has been providing U.S. puffers with highs from the sky."

In his State of the Union message sent to Congress on March 14, 1973, President Nixon said: "One area where I am convinced of the need for immediate action is that of jailing heroin pushers. Under the Bail Reform Act of 1966, a federal judge is precluded from considering the danger to the community when setting bail for suspects arrested for selling heroin. The effect of this restriction is that many accused pushers are immediately released on bail, and are thus given the opportunity to go out and create more misery, generate more violence and commit more crimes while they are waiting to be tried for these same activities.

"This situation is intolerable," President Nixon continued. "I am, therefore, calling upon the Congress to promptly enact a new Heroin Trafficking Act."

Under the new provision, anyone trafficking in less than four ounces of a mixture or substance containing heroin or morphine would receive a mandatory sentence of not less than five years nor more than 15 years. For a first offense of trafficking in four or more ounces of these narcotics, the Act provides a mandatory sentence of not less than 10 years or for life. Those with prior convictions could receive a sentence of from 10 years to life imprisonment—without parole.

"While four ounces of a heroin mixture may seem a very small amount to use as the criterion for major penalties, that amount is actually worth $12,000 to $15,000, and would supply about 180 addicts for a day. Anyone selling four or more ounces cannot be considered a small-time operator," the President said.

Meanwhile, the National Commission on Marijuana and Drug Abuse stated that government efforts may be perpetuating drug use instead of discouraging it. The panel urged creation of a new federal antidrug agency with a limited lifespan and asked private citizens to assume the major burden in discouraging drug use, stated the *New York Post*, March 21, 1973.

"The Commission's sharpest words were aimed at what it called a 'drug-abuse industrial complex,' the welter of federal bureaucracies that now spend nearly $1 billion a year on antidrug programs," the *Post* said.

"To justify ongoing programs, the drug bureaucracy must simultaneously demonstrate that the problem is being effectively attacked and that it is not diminishing. . . . Throughout this process fundamental assumptions are not questioned, programs are not evaluated, and the problem is perpetuated from year to year," the *Post* continued.

The Commission, relatively conservative in makeup, gave the following report to President Nixon and Congress, following a 2-year study:

1) Public notions about drug use are largely wrong.

2) Private citizens rely too much on government to discourage drug use.

3) America's worst drug problem is alcoholism. Heroin is second.

4) Legal use of barbiturate "downers," especially

by housewives is America's hidden drug problem.

5) Marijuana is a minor problem compared to alcohol and other drugs.

On November 1, 1972, Jack Anderson, the syndicated columnist, stated that HEW Secretary Elliot Richardson had "suppressed two controversial drug studies, whose conclusions fly in the face of President Nixon's war on narcotics.

"One startling study, called 'Drug Use and the Youth Culture,' declares boldly that young people use psychedelic drugs for 'a high moral, productive and personality fulfilling purpose'. It suggests that strict law enforcement is also driving young people 'to the left in politics,'" Anderson reported.

The second report, a 3-volume study, "Evaluation of Drug Education Programs," calls the government's drug education efforts misdirected and not helpful, Anderson added. Interviews with more than 150 young drug users in various parts of the U.S. showed that their choices of drugs, in order of popularity, are: alcohol, nicotine, caffeine, marijuana, psychedelics, amphetamines, and to some extent, barbiturates and opiates.

"Drug laws and their enforcement seem to have no effect in deterring the young people we interviewed from illegal drug use," continued Anderson in quoting from the report. "The reasons mainly stem from their common perceptions that drug use is not, or should not be, a criminal act because everybody does it, and because things done to oneself are constitutionally protected. . . . Young people see enforcement as selective enforcement against

them and their preferences. Arrest and prosecution
. . . create a fear and distrust in the youth community, which seems to lead to stronger bonds
among individuals, as they unite against what they
feel is a shared injustice."

The young people interviewed, Anderson said,
felt that they had been singled out, along with
blacks and soldiers in Vietnam, as having *the* drug
problem, yet studies show that other groups, including truck drivers, housewives, doctors, mental patients, etc., seem to be using and abusing drugs to
the same extent that the youngsters are.

In the November 2, 1972 issue of *The New York
Times*, the Department of Health, Education and
Welfare denied that the reports that Jack Anderson
referred to had been locked up. However, the HEW
did release them after Anderson's column appeared.
The studies were made by the Youth Crisis and
Growth Center, New Haven, Conn., and Macro
Systems, Inc., New York City and Silver Springs,
Md.

Stated the *Times*, quoting the report: "In a drug
taking society, many youths choose drugs, especially
marijuana, rather than the adult-accepted and wide-
ly-used alcohol. It does not seem likely that efforts
to stop this kind of 'social' or 'light' drug use will
meet with significant success."

On March 19, 1973, Rep. Bertram L. Podell (D.,
N. Y.) asked for a program of complete heroin
maintenance for narcotic addicts as the best available way to slash the soaring crime rate authorities
attribute to drug addiction. At the same time, Con-

gressman Podell wants a 120-day moratorium on the further expansion of methadone maintenance programs on the grounds that the programs have done great harm by creating a new class of addict.

Added the Congressman: "Methadone, often thought to be a panacea since it carries the government's imprimatur, has compounded the problem and is now the second drug of major abuse. It has fostered multiple drug abuse and created a new generation of addicts—addicts without track marks and with no previous history of heroin addiction. Methadone is not a cure for anything. It is a narcotic and it is dangerous. It can and does kill."

Congressman Podell's study shows that methadone-related deaths in the District of Columbia, Buffalo and Minneapolis exceeded the number of deaths caused by heroin in 1972. In New York, the Poison Control Center showed 250 calls for methadone poisoning in the first four months of 1972, with more than 40 per cent occurring in children aged eight months through five years.

The Congressman's plan would eliminate the addict's need to resort to crime with a program of heroin maintenance. "An available supply of pure heroin would attract addicts as a light attracts moths, with a dramatic drop in drug-related crime as a result," he stated. The cost of maintaining 600,000 addicts on heroin is hundreds of millions of dollars less than current federal expenditures and a savings of billions of dollars now lost in addict-related crimes, he added.

On March 6, 1973, the U.S. Senate passed the

Veterans' Drug and Alcohol Treatment and Rehabilitation Act (S-284). "For the first time in the
VA's history, veterans who have received less than
honorable or general discharges for drug use will
be given help," said Senator Alan Cranston (D.,
Calif.), chairman of the Veterans Affairs Subcommittee on Health and Hospitals, and author of the
bill. "This hits at the hard-core drug-user—the veteran most likely to be forced into crime to support
his drug habit."

Senator Cranston said that the precise numbers of
veterans suffering from drug addiction are not
known, but estimates range from 60,000 to as high
as 400,000.

However, the Defense Department has estimated
that, of 300,000 Army enlisted men who served in
Vietnam between 1970 and 1972, less than 4,000
are civilian drug addicts. Thus, the Pentagon was
trying to dispel a widely held belief that Vietnam
veterans are a major factor in the current heroin
epidemic in the United States. The Pentagon's conclusions are based on a $400,000 government study
by Dr. Lee Robins at Washington University, St.
Louis, Missouri. Dr. Robins said that the purpose
of her study was to determine what happened to
servicemen who used or were exposed to drugs. The
study involved interviews with 13,240 Army enlisted men who returned to the U.S. during September 1971, the height of the so-called "heroin epidemic" among U.S. servicemen in Vietnam.

"Drug addiction among Vietnam veterans, according to the Pentagon, is running about 1.3 per cent,

which corresponds closely to the rate of drug users found among youths examined for military service," stated *The New York Times*, April 24, 1973. "The conclusion drawn by the Defense Department was that the exposure of Army men to drugs while in Vietnam had not significantly added to the drug addiction rate found among the civilian population."

Dr. Richard S. Wilbur, Assistant Secretary of Defense for Health and Environment, said that probably not more than 2,000 to 3,000 servicemen who served between 1970 and 1972 are now drug-dependent.

Dr. Robins' study showed that the man most likely to have been a drug user in Vietnam was young, single, a low-ranking member of the regular Army with little education, who came from a broken home, had an arrest history before enlisting and had used drugs before military service.

"One result of the study, Dr. Wilbur observed, is to explode a 'myth' that drug abusers in Vietnam were 'highly deviant men' who were unable to overcome their dependence on drugs," the *Times* said.

"*Licit and Illicit Drugs*, by Edward M. Beecher and the editors of *Consumer Reports* (published by Little, Brown 1972, $12.50), is an exhaustive study that has been five years in preparation," stated the December 2, 1972 issue of *Science News*. "In 70 chapters the report gives historical perspective and up-to-date research findings on each of the classes of drugs in its subtitle: 'narcotics, stimulants, depressants, inhalants, hallucinogens and marijuana —including caffeine, nicotine and alcohol.'

"The report's central theme is the physicians' maxim: *Nihil nocere*. It means that a physician must guard against doing more harm than good. Some particular anti-drug prescriptions are warned against:

"1) Stop emphasizing measures designed to keep drugs away from people. Prohibition pushes prices and crime rates up. It causes users to change from relatively bland, bulky substances to readily smugglable, more hazardous concentrates.

"2) Stop publicizing the horrors of the 'drug menace.' Sensationalist publicity is ineffective and counterproductive. Almost no one had heard of (glue sniffing) in 1959, when a *Denver Post* headline proclaimed 'some glues are dangerous—heavy inhalation can cause anemia or brain damage.' Within 26 months, the Denver Juvenile Court was averaging 30 cases a month of glue sniffing. The publicity and the problem spread across the country.

"3) Stop increasing the damage done by drugs. Current drug laws make drugs more rather than less dangerous. For instance, the sale or possession of hypodermic needles without prescription is a criminal offense. This leads to non-sterile needles, the sharing of needles and then to epidemics of hepatitis and other needle-borne diseases. . . .

"4) Stop misclassifying drugs. Illogical and capricious classification of drugs destroys credibility. The report calls for distinctions between more hazardous and less hazardous drugs, instead of between licit and illicit drugs.

"5) Stop pursuing the goal of stamping out illicit

drug use. Efforts to stamp out one drug shift users to another drug," *Science News* reported.

Impotency is closely related to drug addiction, according to Dr. Alan J. Cooper of London. He said, "Of recent interest and importance is doctor-induced impotence following the use of certain medications. These include a wide range of addictive drugs, the best known of which is probably alcohol. Other drugs capable of causing impotence (a loss of sexual powers, especially among males) include anti-depressants and tranquilizers. Suffice it to say there are at present over 20 medicines widely prescribed which are capable of depriving a male of his masculinity."

Some drug addicts, when they give up heroin in exchange for methadone, become alcoholics, according to the April 14, 1973 issue of *Science News*.

"Doctors at the Baltimore City Hospital used the reinforcing properties of methadone to get alcoholic patients to take disulfiram (Antabuse), an alcohol antagonist. The patients were given methadone only if they took disulfiram. As expected, alcoholism was controlled. But the researchers admit in the April *American Journal of Psychiatry* that 'disulfiram will not affect the causes of these patients' drinking any more than methadone treatment gets at the roots of heroin addiction," *Science News* stated.

At the 57th annual meeting of the Federation of American Societies for Experimental Biology, held in April 1973 in Atlantic City, New Jersey, scientists at the University of Pittsburgh reported that a natural body chemical injected into experimental animals had dramatically reversed the effects of overdoses of such depressants as barbiturates and alcohol.

"The scientists raised the possibility that synthetic preparations of this chemical—called cyclic AMP— might someday be used in man to counter the effects of barbiturate abuse and of alcohol misuse, if it can be shown that this use of the chemical would be safe," reported *The New York Times,* April 17, 1973.

Six medical doctors, all at the College of Physicians and Surgeons, Columbia University, cautioned that marijuana should not be made available commercially in the United States, as has been suggested by the National Organization for the Reform of Marijuana Laws and others. Writing in the May 31, 1973 issue of *The New York Times,* Drs. Robert E. Esser, Henry Clay Frick II, Albert Greenwood, Gabriel G. Nahas, Phillip Zeidenberg and William M. Manger listed many ways in which marijuana can be harmful: marijuana contains toxic substances (THC and its metabolites); moderate usage is difficult to achieve and the user generally escalates to more potent drugs; marijuana smoke induces cancer in tissue cultures of human lungs; marijuana usage leads to cellular damage in man; etc.

CHAPTER 7

Prescribed and Over-the-Counter Drugs Are a Threat to Your Nutritional Health

At a December 5, 1972 hearing on drug abuse, in Washington, Senator Gaylord Nelson (D., Wis.) said that, in 1969, the public spent nearly $1 billion on cough and cold remedies, tablets, capsules, drops and sprays. Senator Nelson described these medicines as "mostly useless and sometimes even dangerous."

The Wisconsin Senator added that we want a pill for every ache and pain, for nervous tension, for anxiety and even for the ordinary stresses and strains of daily living. "In short," he said, "we have become massively addicted to taking drugs whether we need them or not. The result is that we have created a drug culture and many of the youth of America are simply doing what they have learned from their parents."

It is readily apparent that Americans have a nationwide preoccupation with drugs of many kinds, some of them non-addicting, most of them very definitely addictive. Much of this addiction has originated in doctor's offices, where tranquilizers, pep pills and all manner of other mood-altering drugs are given almost routinely for patients who are troublesome or seem to have complaints for which there is no organic reason. Almost no effort is ever made to determine what daily habits of the complaining patient may be responsible for the symptoms: diet, lack of sleep, boredom, lack of exercise, lack of fresh air or clean water, noise pollution, to name a few.

It's easier for the doctor and takes much less time to hand over a bottle of tranquilizers and sleeping pills, "diet pills" for the overweight, mood-altering pills for the depressed patient. The idea of ever prescribing such drugs for children seems outrageous, yet it is being done through the school physician in some localities. Aspirin, the king of self-medications, can be very toxic, especially among children. It can erode away the lining of the stomach and thus cause ulcers.

More than 200 million prescriptions for psychoactive drugs, most of them to alleviate anxiety, frustration, agitation and depression, are filled annually, despite our knowledge that they do not erase everyday problems. Nor do we know the immediate or long-range consequences of these drugs, according to an article in the September 1971 issue of the *Illinois Medical Journal*.

A recent article in the *Ladies Home Journal* reviewed the experiences of 4,000 New York women —a survey which is believed to be representative of women all over the country. Results showed that 25 per cent of all women interviewed had taken drugs to relax them; 37 per cent had taken "noncontrolled narcotics;" 22 per cent had taken barbiturates; 8 per cent had used marijuana; 17 per cent had used "diet pills" (amphetamines are the most common of these); 9 per cent had taken non-barbiturate sedatives; 6 per cent had taken pep pills; 4 per cent "anti-depressants;" 2 per cent had experimented with LSD; 8 per cent had taken "controlled narcotics" (opium, Demarol, morphine, etc.); 3 per cent had taken major tranquilizers (the anti-depressants); and 2 per cent had used other hallucinogenic drugs.

Almost all of these women had obtained the tranquilizers from their doctors, although one in 25 reported that she did not always use them as the doctor had recommended. Three out of every 20 women who use sleeping pills regularly said they got them from sources other than doctors. Forty per cent admitted that they use these addictive drugs in ways their doctors do not recommend. Thirty eight per cent of those who use "pep pills" do not get them from doctors. College co-eds take the highest risks, it seems.

In February 1972, the Food and Drug Administration announced that it was cutting the production quota for amphetamines to about 17-18 per cent of the 1971 quota, "in an effort to cope with one of the nation's most serious drug problems." It is estimated that about 20 per cent of all these "pep pills" have been diverted into illegal channels. Addicts use them to produce "highs." Long-distance truck drivers use them to stay awake so they can somehow manage to make the impossible schedules they must meet. Improper use of these drugs is considered extremely dangerous and has led to deaths, not to mention traffic accidents.

"The currently accepted primary medical uses of the amphetamines and their related compounds are in treating two conditions—narcolepsy and a hyperactivity disorder among children," according to the FDA. Narcolepsy, an uncommon disorder, is an excessive tendency to sleep. Hyperactivity among children is considered fairly common. But only some of these children respond to treatment by amphetamines. Vitamin therapy, as we will discover in another chapter, is generally much wiser.

The New York Times for January 16, 1973 told the story of a New York physician who treats many rich and famous people, keeping them addicted to amphetamines and other drugs which he injects. The patients are apparently completely dependent upon these injections, which give them such "highs" that they talk incessantly and feel fine until the effects wear off. Then they begin to have withdrawal symptoms. Thus, they have to get another injection.

Other doctors are apparently unwilling or unable to do anything about the situation. When they try to treat these patients, the victims themselves insist that they be allowed to return to the doctor who gives them "the magic shots."

The New York County Medical Society said that they are powerless to discipline any physician unless his patients bring charges. Doctors who were interviewed by *The New York Times* had not filed any complaints against the doctor who had purportedly been too free in his use of the pep pills, because, apparently, of reasons involving "medical ethics."

The New York City doctor who gives these drugs, who now faces indictment, had accompanied President Kennedy to a Summit meeting in 1961 and had given him injections of amphetamines then and also just before a speech at the United Nations. Said the *Times*, "The fact that a physician . . . could treat—without the public's knowledge—a Commander-in-Chief who holds the power to use atomic weapons and make decisions that affect the political health of the world raises anew the question of a need for full disclosure of the President's medical record."

One doctor said, in reply to the *Times* article, "If all drugs which are being abused 'by unqualified users' would be removed from medical practice, therapy would be set back at least 100 years."

In Canada, the use of amphetamines has been sharply restricted. Any physician prescribing them for a patient must give the federal health department the name of his patient. If the drug is to be used for longer than 30 days, he must also give the name of another doctor who has examined the patient. Many Canadians are already dependent on one or more of this family of drugs, said a spokesman of the Canadian Medical Association.

In 1970, there were horrifying reports of 3,000 to 6,000 students in Omaha schools who were being given "behavior drugs" to improve their conduct and learning ability. The amphetamines were being used, along with other tranquilizers to "help" hyperactive children who are restless, overactive, with short attention spans. The cause of the condition is not known, said *Newsweek*, commenting on the incident. One doctor stated that children are inattentive because they are bored and tired. Amphetamines seem to help by increasing alertness and relieving fatigue. It seems to us that fatigue can be relieved only with rest.

At any rate, many mothers of the drugged children were understandably concerned lest their children come to believe that, later in life, popping a pill is the answer to any problem or trauma. Why not? Isn't a dependence on amphetamines, begun in grade school, almost a guarantee that the taker will be addicted to these pills or some substitute for them later in life?

At a 1972 Senate hearing on drugs, three medical experts expressed doubt that the public would ever give up its "diet pills." Dr. Jean Mayer of Harvard, an authority on obesity, said that "in the case of amphetamines, the limited usefulness to some patients does not counterbalance the enormous social cost brought about by the availability of pep pills." And Dr. Jay Tepperman, Professor of Experimental Medicine at the Upstate Medical Center in Syracuse, said: "Fat people are very interesting to pharmaceutical manufacturers because there are so many of them."

Dr. Thaddeus E. Prout of the Greater Baltimore Medical Center said that the AMA is abetting the use of diet pills by not exerting its influence to stop the practice. Drug companies pour some 12 million dollars in advertising into AMA publications. They have persuaded the AMA to disband its Council on Drugs, which for many years had been very critical of the "irrational" use of such drugs as reducing pills.

On April 1, 1973, the Bureau of Narcotics and Dangerous Drugs and the Food and Drug Administration in Washington announced that they would recall diet drugs that contain amphetamines, with the objective of eliminating them from the marketplace by June 30. The action is designed to end the use of all injectable amphetamine, and closely related chemicals, and all combinations of diet pills that contain amphetamine and other ingredients, such as vitamins or a sedative, stated *The New York Times*, April 2, 1973.

Controlled substances are prescription drugs that can be dispensed only with special safeguards such as nonrefillable prescriptions and extra record-keeping obligations on the part of the doctor, the *Times* said.

"The decision to recall existing stocks of the injectable amphetamines is based on the FDA's contention that these products have such a great drug abuse potential that they cannot be used safely," the *Times* continued. "The agency considers the combination drugs, taken by mouth, to be ineffective on

110

the grounds that the amphetamines do little good in obesity control and the other ingredients contribute nothing useful toward this objective."

In the three months following the recall order, between 10,000 and 20,000 retail and wholesale outlets were visited by federal and state officers to insure that the drugs were taken out of circulation. The amphetamines make up the bulk of the diet pill market, with yearly retail distribution estimated at about 480 million dosage units—equivalent to that many 10 mg. pills.

The drug recall notice, published in the *Federal Register*, makes it unlawful, with a few exceptions, to ship any of the combination pills or the injectable amphetamines in interstate commerce. The injectable products to be banned include not only amphetamine itself, but also dextroamphetamine, levamphetamine and methamphetamine, all related substances.

The exceptions, noted the *Times*, are several products of manufacturers who, at the time of this writing, have asked for hearings before the FDA. These products are Obetrol-10 and Obetrol-20 tablets, manufactured by a division of Rexer Pharmacal Corp., Brooklyn, New York; Eskatrol Spansules, Dexamyl tablets, Elixir and Spansules of Smith, Kline & French Laboratories, Philadelphia, Pennsylvania; Bamadex Sequels of Lederle Laboratories Division of American Cyanamid, Pearl River, New York; and Delcobese tablets, sustained release tablets, capsules and sustained release capsules of Delco Chemical, Mount Vernon, New York.

"All of those products may continue to be marketed pending a ruling on the requests for hearings before the FDA," the *Times* added. "Although some of these, such as Dexamyl, are among the most widely used of the combination drugs, the total impact of these exceptions is small, considering that there are about 1,500 products involved altogether. The combination products are estimated to make up 72 per cent of all the appetite suppressing drugs prescribed by doctors."

In spite of the recall, the FDA still considers the amphetamines, used alone, to have some legitimate usefulness as a short-term aid to the treatment of obesity. However, the agency warns doctors that the drugs should be prescribed and dispensed sparingly, and that they should be used for only a short time on those patients who have not had any weight reduction under other programs.

In a recent issue of *Science* (the publication of the American Association for the Advancement of Science) two letters to the editor speak about the use of medicinal drugs in this country. A representative of the Pharmaceutical Manufacturers Association tells *Science* readers that, while there are many Americans who use lots of drugs constantly or occasionally, there are also a large number of people who should be taking drugs who never do, because they neglect their health or because they can't afford drugs, or because they just fail to get prescriptions filled or because they seem to feel that there is something gallant about enduring unnecessary pain, or because they have been educated to believe that taking medicinal drugs is equated with personal failings.

Says this gentleman, quoting a study by the National Institutes of Health. "This study clearly contradicts the labeling of our society as 'overmedicated.' He goes on to say that doctors are not 'overprescribing' and challenges the concept that drugs can be proven to be 'safe' or 'superior' to other drugs already in use. He praises the use of drugs since they have saved lives, aborted or relieved illnesses, shortened hospital stays and saved time lost from work."

The other letter deals with "the appalling amount of sickness" which the conscientious physician sees all about him. "There is very good argument," he says, "for the fact that our society is undermedicated." Physicians are so busy and they lack any kind of paramedical help, so, he says, they tend to look the other way when disease stares them in the face. "In the process of taking the proper corrective measures, we shall soon see what every honest doctor knows. There is currently not enough medicine available to help all the sick people in our society if we earnestly set about trying to help them," he says.

The health seeker, on the other hand, accustomed to looking for the real causes of illness, is baffled by this point of view among doctors. Apparently, they believe—or most of them believe—that illness is a mysterious something that falls from the sky and afflicts this or that patient arbitrarily. Nothing he can do will affect the course of the disease except to take drugs. And so carefully has the medical profession promoted this concept that many people actually do ask their doctor for miracle drugs rather than seeking his advice on how they might change their lives to be more healthy.

Almost never does an article in a medical journal recommend daily outdoor exercise as a treatment for many chronic disorders. Almost never does a medical journal speak of proper diet and enough pure water as the single most important factor separating poor health from abundant good health.

Almost never, if one can believe the medical journals, does a doctor even ask his patient what he has been eating all his life—even when the disease is intimately involved with diet, such as diabetes and digestive diseases. Apparently, it never occurs to the average doctor that the only things which ever get inside his patients are air, water and food, along with those toxic pollutants which are unavoidable in our industrial society.

So whole families, addicted to sleeping pills, tranquilizers, pep pills, reducing pills, pain pills, produce youngsters who become addicted to heroin, LSD, marijuana, alcohol or nicotine. Weren't they brought up to believe that drugs are the universal panacea?

How can we get our population back on the way to true health? By continuing to insist to our congressmen, our health officials, our doctors, our educators that the healthy body does *not* get sick and the only way to have a healthy body is to observe for a whole lifetime those rules for a sound, wholesome, nutritious diet, good pure water, fresh air, plenty of invigorating outdoor exercise, stimulating, meaningful work and truly restful relaxation.

Let's encourage this kind of health rather than the drug-oriented kind, which isn't real health, after all. Even the Olympic Games are not immune from drugs. The November 10, 1972 issue of *The New York Times* carried an article, "Use of Drugs at Olympics Found to Be Widespread." Said the *Times:* Despite elaborate doping control procedures, the use and availability of drugs at the recent Olympics appear to have been the most widespread and open in the history of the modern games."

An Australian physician believes that patients in intensive care in hospitals should be given prophylactic doses of vitamin K, according to *Medical World News* for June 16, 1972. Dr. John Ham says that such patients may have disordered blood clotting reactions because of the way they are being maintained in the hospital. They may have trouble with liver or gall bladder, which might interfere with the vitamin's absorption. Perhaps they are not getting enough of it in the hospital diet, or their intestinal bacteria may not be able to manufacture it, as the bacteria do in a healthy digestive tract.

Vitamin K is a neglected element in our official thinking about nutrition. *Recommended Dietary Allowances* says, "Because of lack of reliable information concerning human intakes of vitamin K and because of other factors shown to be operative in experimental animals, but not yet evaluated in man, an absolute daily allowance for this vitamin has not been established." Non-prescription vitamin supplements are not permitted to include the vitamin, since pregnant women supposedly might get too much of it for the welfare of their babies during childbirth.

This story gives us a hint of the many factors which are involved which endanger our access to vitamins. Drugs are among the most threatening of these. Did you know that your nutritional state may be greatly influenced by the drugs you take, that many drugs actually destroy vitamins and minerals in your body while others may react with one another or with food to produce astonishing, uncomfortable, perhaps fatal effects?

In the January 1968 issue of the *Journal of the American Dietetic Association*, two New York physicians write about the inter-relationships of diets and drugs. They say that patients who consult their doctor about some disease that affects nutritional status may not know that the drug he gives them may affect what goes on in their bodies in relation to food. Or he may have to prescribe some kind of diet for their condition—and this too may change their nutritional status.

A low-sodium diet, for instance, may be prescribed for high blood pressure or edema. If the person has been accustomed to large amounts of salt, he may find his food almost inedible without it. So he may become badly nourished just from not eating a full diet. People with extremely high cholesterol levels are often put on diets in which animal fat is reduced to a minimum and the patient is told to eat lots of vegetable oils—that is, salad oils. He may find such a diet unpalatable and he also may become short in vitamin E, since this vitamin is related to the amount of unsaturated fat in one's food.

If the individual is told to eat a low fat diet, he is likely to lack vitamin A and the other fat-soluble vitamins. If he must go on a high-fat diet, he is almost certain to end up with high levels of cholesterol. If the doctor puts him on a diet consisting mostly of protein, the patient's requirement for one of the B vitamins, pyridoxine, is greatly increased. If one's condition necessitates a high carbohydrate diet, one is likely to become deficient in thiamine (vitamin B1).

On the other hand, certain diseases and conditions of ill health have a definite effect on the nutriment that is available for one. People who are almost immobile in bed for even quite short periods of time lose calcium and nitrogen in their urine. Cancer patients are frequently treated with drugs which destroy certain vitamins. They may also lack appetite and hence become deficient in vitamins and minerals.

People with chronic disorders of the digestive tract suffer from lack of appetite, nausea, losses of many nutrients through vomiting and diarrhea. Many people suffer from chronic diarrhea which means that they do not absorb many things in their food. They may eventually become quite deficient in protein, vitamins and minerals. Kidney disease patients lose protein in their urine.

Now let us look at the effects of some drugs on

essential nutrients. If you take antacid preparations for an ulcer, you will likely be short on thiamine, for it is rapidly destroyed in an alkaline medium. Mineral oil dissolves and renders ineffective all the fat-soluble vitamins—A, D, E and K. Chelating agents which are given for certain conditions absorb metals, that is minerals, so that they are not available to your body. Resins which are given as drugs in some conditions unbalance your body's supplies of sodium, potassium and calcium, three important minerals.

Drugs called anti-metabolites, which are given for certain quite serious conditions, destroy folic acid, which prevents a form of anemia. Barbiturates and anticonvulsant drugs given in disorders like epilepsy also destroy folic acid. Corticosteroids such as ACTH and cortisone may cause diabetes by disturbing the blood sugar regulating mechanism, may produce loss of potassium, may cause ulcers.

What about the antibiotics—those life-saving wonder drugs which fight infections? They may, because of their composition, have a direct action on the digestive tract, resulting in diarrhea, nausea, loss of appetite and mouth irritation. Penicillin, the sulfa drugs and chloromycetin may disturb the body's use of protein, thus creating many kinds of future difficulties.

Tetracycline, another antibiotic, may affect the calcium in bones. Isoniazid, used to treat tuberculosis, may destroy vitamin B6. The sulfa drugs attack the friendly bacteria in the digestive tract which may eventually produce troublesome digestive disorders and may result in lack of vitamin K and some B vitamins which these bacteria synthesize. Neomycin may cause such an upset in the digestive tract that vitamin A, vitamin B12, cholesterol and sugar may not be properly absorbed.

Now we come to the most serious part of taking drugs—especially combinations of drugs which is a common practice these days. Certain diuretics cause the body to lose potassium, a mineral. If the patient is taking digitalis at the same time—and this is just the kind of patient who might be—the toxic effects of the digitalis are increased. The heart may begin to flutter and beat in a most irregular way. Then there is a group of new drugs called by the jaw-breaking name of monoamine oxidase inhibitors. One of these is an antidepressant drug which is often given to mentally ill patients. Only recently it was discovered that, if the patient taking these drugs eats a piece of cheese, or liver, certain kinds of beans or a piece of herring, or if he has even one drink, he is likely to experience terrifying symptoms, including severe headache, sudden high blood pressure, changes in heart rate, sweating, nausea, vomiting, and, in some cases, death from stroke. Now the drug itself does not produce these symptoms. It is only when the patient eats certain foods which contain substances that react with the drug that the symptoms are produced.

Undoubtedly, new drugs developed in future years will produce many more such tales to tell. It almost makes you vow never to take another drug.

Before we leave the subject of drugs, we would like to quote Nicholas Johnson, Commissioner of the Federal Communications Commission, who recently appeared at a hearing held by the National Council of Churches on "Patterns of Drug Use and Misuse in American Society." The meeting was held in Washington.

"We've got a drug problem in America," he said. "It's called television. During my term as an FCC Commissioner I have often appeared before committees of the United States Senate and the House of Representatives, and various concerned citizens' groups with this message. And yet, if there has been any change in either the marketing use of drugs in this nation during the past six years, it has been a change for the worse. . . .

"When you realize that television has such an enormous impact upon our behavior patterns, and that it is the advertising industry, in conjunction with its corporate clients, which has been given unchecked power to dictate what an entire nation will be permitted to watch on the tube, you have begun to comprehend the problem of broadcasting in our society.

"Naturally," Commissioner Johnson continued, "several of the advertising industry's clients are drug manufacturers. These manufacturers, like the other producers who thrive on the consumption ethic in this nation, barrage us daily with their message. They, like du Pont, tell us incessantly that we can achieve 'better living through chemistry'. . . .

Though their message is brought to us primarily through advertisements, America's drug manufacturers have (conveyed) that message through other, often more insidious means. . . .

"Alcohol gets a very sympathetic endorsement from Big Broadcasting in both commercials and programs. Beer and wine are pushed openly and hard. It's as if television were committed to stamping out the use of protein as an energy source. While the little kids are being told the lie that strength comes from sugar and cereal flakes robbed of almost all their natural nutritional value, and sugar-coated vitamins that look and taste like candy, their teenage brothers and sisters are being told the lie that beer will give them 'gusto'—as well as sexuality, acceptability and all the material things in life for which they yearn. . . .

"Rather than charge for the hard liquor commercials, TV gives them away—as well it can afford to. Beer and wine commercials brought broadcasters $105 million last year—and that figure only covers TV (not radio), and only national—not local—advertising. Drinking and alcoholism are seldom, if ever, given serious treatment on television. Drunks are frequently portrayed as comedy characters. Alcoholics Anonymous is sometimes the butt of demeaning jokes. What is worse, TV personalities who are widely revered . . . actually make heavy drinking a major element in the lovable-full-of-life fun characters they play. Story lines of programs often include someone with a problem turning, almost casually, to a drink of alcohol as a solution. Drinking is almost always associated with social sophistication and acceptability.

"In short," Commissioner Johnson said, "television, its advertising agencies, and their corporate clients are preying upon both our minds and our bodies—and those of defenseless children—to promote atheistic corporate greed whatever the social cost."

Commissioner Johnson quotes Art Linkletter, the entertainer, who is President of the National Coordinating Council of Drug Education, and who was speaking before the United Nations General Assembly in 1971.

Said Mr. Linkletter, whose child died from an overdose of LSD: "Advertisements in the mass media cajole us into believing that there is a pill for every ill . . . real or imagined. Doctors, pharmacists and drug manufacturers have reinforced our hope that relief from any kind of anxiety is only a swallow away . . . four out of five adults use some kind of mood-inducing chemical regularly: nicotine, alcohol, caffeine, amphetamines for a pick-up . . . and in the last few years, hallucinogens of every imaginable type to shut out the grim reality and transport us to a fantasy dream world. With this as a model, is it any surprise that our young people have turned to drugs in ever increasing numbers?" Linkletter said.

CHAPTER 8

Some Reasons Why So Many Children and Adults Are Hooked on Drugs and Sugar

"THE EDUCATIONAL ATTEMPTS that have been made in the areas of drug abuse, alcoholism, prevention of heart attacks and smoking have not been very encouraging. What about trying to educate for optimal nutritional health as a preventive measure to these problems? Possibly, if our population were adequately fed through making good choices according to their own knowledge, there would be less desire for changing one's health through various kinds of abuses." This was part of the prepared statement by Dr. George M. Briggs, Professor of Nutrition, Department of Nutritional Sciences, University of California, Berkeley, and Helen D. Ullrich, M.A., R.D., editor of the *Journal of Nutrition Education*. They were appearing at hearings of the

U. S. Senate Select Committee on Nutrition and Human Needs in Washington on December 5, 1972.

We have already noted throughout this book some of the abuses that can affect our health. At a Conference on the Medical Complications of Drug Abuse, presented by the American Medical Association in December 1972 in New York, it was pointed out that the causes of death among heroin addicts are generally attributed first to overdoses, then to suicide, homicide or other trauma, then to medical complications of heroin use. Their nutritional status was not mentioned, but we can assume that it was quite poor.

"Ninety per cent of all tetanus cases in New York City are addicts, Charles Cherubin of Metropolitan Hospital, New York, reported," said the December 16, 1972 issue of *Science News*. "The tetanus is apparently caused by skin popping and using a quinine solution of heroin. Although there is virtually no malaria among addicts in the eastern United States, because they put heroin in quinine, 50 cases of malaria have been diagnosed among addicts in California. Apparently, they don't use quinine. About a third to one-half of all addicts get hepatitis from dirty needles. Fifty per cent of all newborns born to addicts have hepatitis. Alcohol can complicate heroin-induced hepatitis by making the liver deteriorate three or four times faster."

Continued *Science News:* "'We are presently studying street heroin material,' said John Sheagren of the District of Columbia General Hospital. So far he and his team have cultured 31 harmful microorganisms from the material. 'Fever in addicts,' he asserted, 'is all that is needed to suspect deep-seated, life-threatening infection.'

"A. I. Weidman of New York University School of Medicine and his colleagues have examined the skin of 1,000 addicts and have noted skin abcesses, ulcers, edema, hyperpigmentation. One addict, Weidman said, injected his fingers so many times they would no longer bend. Another addict ran out of veins and started injecting himself in the penis.

" 'Addicts,' the article continued, " 'are using not only quinine, but sucrose (sugar), baking soda, aspirin, atrophine and strychina as dilutants for heroin,' Weidman pointed out. Addicts are also mixing penicillin with heroin, 'which may create a new clinical syndrome,' asserted J. Willis Hurst of the Emory University School of Medicine."

The conference was also told that contaminants from heroin, from the solution it is in or from the cotton it is filtered through can circulate through the blood and lodge in capillaries of the lung.

Stated Ralph Richter of the Harlem Hospital Center: "The cerebral complications that can result from heroin overdose include coma, seizures, deafness, stroke and brain damage." He told of one patient who took 50 bags of heroin in one day and lost most of the vision in one of his eyes.

With all of these grim statistics being repeated in virtually every city in the nation, how and why do so many children get hooked on drugs? Undoubtedly, there is a considerable element of daring and status-seeking involved. If the other kids are doing it, if it's the thing to do, many children—especially those with little or no parental supervision and those who are least secure in their relationships with others—will have to try it so they can boast of their daring exploit.

But this still does not explain the addiction. Why, after they have tried one or several drugs, the novelty has worn off and they have established their place in the young peoples' community, are so many of them caught up in true addiction from which they cannot escape?

We suggest the reason is that many of them have been addicted since the cradle or the playpen —addicted to that insidious drug whose use is so widespread in this country and other developed nations of the world. We refer to sugar, which for many people is as truly addictive as any other drug. In his fine book, *Dr. Atkins' Diet Revolution,* Dr. Robert C. Atkins, who has made a lifelong study of what sugar does to susceptible people, says: "Addictive people seem to have one thing in common: an underlying hypoglycemia (low blood sugar). We certainly see hypoglycemia in sugar addicts, in alcoholics, in coffee addicts. People who have studied hard-drug addicts report to me that hypoglycemia is common among them. Cola beverages have long been addictive for many people.

"The starches can be addictive, too," says Dr. Atkins. "Many forms of the starches can be addictive, though this is somewhat less common. Potato chips. Bread. Crackers. Pizzas. Spaghetti. And when refined flour is combined with refined sugar, as in cakes, pies, cookies, desserts, only a tiny bit is required to set the whole vicious cycle in motion again."

The pervasive influence of soft drinks in this area of American life may surprise you. Did you know many babies are started off on cola drinks almost from the moment of birth? In Senator George McGovern's 1969 hearings on food and nutrition, one member of the committee, Senator Talmadge of Georgia, asked the president of Coca-Cola:

"I know in some circles Coca-Cola is considered to be of high nutritional value. . . . When my oldest son was born, the pediatrician prescribed Coca-Cola for our infant son. Is that a common practice?"

And the president of Coca-Cola replied:

"It is common practice by pediatricians throughout the country, and of long standing, and the question is repeatedly asked, 'Why doesn't the company publicize this?' We have a stock answer and that is we would rather have it by word-of-mouth among pediatricians rather than departing from the company's attitude that we sell a soft drink which has delicious, refreshing qualities and that only."

We wrote to the American Medical Association, the National Institutes of Health and the American Academy of Pediatrics to inquire why anyone should give babies Coca-Cola and why Coca-Cola should be prescribed in many hospitals.

The National Institutes of Health told us they have no idea why doctors should prescribe soft drinks. The Institutes have no official position on this question, they added. And they enclosed a leaflet on nutrition, just in case we might need this general information.

The scientific Director of the National Institute of Child Health and Human Development wrote us that many pediatricians use Coca-Cola "as a digestive" for infants. "I know of no scientific basis for this practice," their spokesman said, "and remain uncertain whether it serves any useful purpose."

The head of the Committee on Nutrition of the American Academy of Pediatrics told us that it is "common practice" among pediatricians to give Coca-Cola to infants who have digestive upsets with vomiting. They believe that the phosphoric acid in the coke is beneficial. A drug firm, in fact, markets a form of this phosphoric acid to relieve vomiting. "I suspect," he went on, "that much of the benefit of Coke . . . resides with the fact that the mother feels she is doing something about the child's vomiting by offering small sips of a solution which will be retained. Whether or not one can ascribe an anti-emetic effect to . . . syrup of Coca-Cola might be difficult to establish by appropriate clinical study."

He refers to "syrup of Coca-Cola" since, he tells us, some baby specialists advise mothers to purchase the straight Coke syrup as it is dispensed at the soda fountain. This must be almost entirely sugar, along with any of the nearly 1,000 chemical additives which are at present legally permitted in all soft drinks.

The American Medical Association wrote us that cokes and other carbonated beverages "have become so popular among us that they are part of our society and consequently they effect (sic) our psyche. People are so use (sic) to them that when illness strikes them many are willing to drink soft drinks rather than other conventional foods or juices. *(Ed. If that isn't addiction, what is?)* This explains the wide use of soft drinks for forcing fluids, nausea, digestive problems, etc. . . . However, there is no scientific evidence that carbonated beverages aid in digestion, prevents (sic) nausea, etc. . . . Consumption of soft drinks by the healthy individual is all right as long as they do not replace foods that are necessary for proper nutrition. The ingredients in soft drinks have been approved by the FDA. That means they are safe for human consumption."

By now close to $5 billion a year are spent by Americans for soft drinks. Dr. Henry Schroeder of Dartmouth Medical School tells us that he inquired of the Pepsi-Cola Company about individual consumption. He was told the "average" American drinks about nine bottles of soft drinks per day.

"If the above is correct," he continues, "it is obvious that the Average American no longer goes to the tap to quench his thirst but opens a bottle." Apparently the American Medical Association, which continues to tell us that soft drinks do no harm as long as they do not replace other more nutritious beverages, has never heard that the average American has just about stopped drinking any beverage but soft drinks.

If, indeed, the average consumption is nine bottles a day, there are certainly thousands of people who are forbidden by their doctors to use soft drinks, so the people who really *do* drink them must be drinking far more than nine bottles a day. What room does that leave in the stomach of a small child for fruit juices and milk?

Slightly more than half of all soft drinks consumed are colas. The cola drinks contain caffeine—a substance which is just as harmful to the body regulatory mechanism for sugar when it occurs in soft drinks as it is when it appears in coffee. A recent syndicated medical column in the daily paper carried a question from an anxious mother. She said: "My son used to be an alcoholic. Since he reformed he has become a coffee addict; he drinks it day and night. Is there a cure for this addiction?" The doctor's answer: "Be satisfied for the present. One peep out of you about coffee and your son may return to alcohol. The basic cause of many habits and addictions is the same. A person addicted to one drug often switches to another. Coffee overindulgence is one of the least harmful habits."

There seems to be little doubt that many alcoholics throughout the world are almost immediately addicted to coffee as soon as they manage to shake off the chains of addiction to alcohol. The coffee urn bubbles and steams at drying-out centers and social centers for drug addicts. Sugar is free and the truly addicted personality is likely to load his coffee with three or four teaspoons of the sweet, white stuff, which produces, just for a little while, almost the same calming effect as the drug he is attempting to free himself from. Blood sugar levels leap up. That jittery, "lost" feeling calms down, the butterflies in the stomach go away. For a short time.

Drinking caffeine-rich beverages on an empty stomach has a more deleterious effect than drinking them with food—just the same as alcohol and cigarettes. In addition, there seems to be some evidence that drinking caffeine in a *cold* beverage has a more powerful effect on the body than if the beverage is hot. So on these two counts alone, soft drinks may be more dangerous and more addictive than coffee.

But the children in this century don't just drink soft drinks as one of the major elements in their diets. Available today on every side, everywhere you go, are other inexpensive, high-carbohydrate foods: potato chips, candy, crackers, cookies, cupcakes, doughnuts, pastries, cakes, pies, chewing gum, sundaes and an almost endless variety of snack foods which contain almost nothing but carbohydrate—plus the additives, preservatives, synthetic dyes and flavorings which are essential to make these foods palatable and to keep them unspoiled on store shelves and in dispensers until they are sold.

Schools find that many children may forego the school lunch and spend their lunch money on potato chips, cokes and candy. In fact, some school administrators use this as an excuse for continuing to sell goodies in the school lunchroom. Everywhere else that children go, from the moment they are able to walk, they are plied with sugary goodies by kindly relatives, friends and neighbors. Banks and doctors' offices present any child who enters with a lollipop. Supermarkets place candy machines at the check-out counter so that, while mother is paying the bill, the kids beg for a few coins and get another sugary snack to keep them going on the way home. Any holiday occasion is another excuse for such an orgy of sweets; they go home surfeited and stuffed. And, of course, they don't have room to eat whatever nutritious, high-protein food may be offered them at the evening meal.

As a result, the incidence of obesity and overweight among children is rising to alarming levels. It appears that the fat child is bound to become the fat adult with very special problems of overcoming that condition, which the thin child does not have.

How much drug addiction among youngsters is caused directly by the amount of sugar they have eaten during their childhood is impossible to know. However, nutritional surveys conducted by the U. S. Department of Agriculture and the U. S. Public Health Service have shown that the poor eating habits resulting in malnutrition are common, not just among poor people who cannot afford the higher-priced, high-protein food. Many middle-income and upper-income families eat totally unbalanced meals, often at irregular hours. Skipping breakfast has become so common among children that many schools are now providing breakfast as well as lunch for those children who can afford breakfast at home, as well as those who cannot.

When one reads of the near miraculous treatment of drug addiction with diet and megadoses of vitamins, one wonders why, while our health officials have bewailed our mounting addiction figures, and spent astronomical sums of money investigating supposedly every aspect of it, not a single public official has ever connected addiction with a national diet deficient in many essential nutrients and overflowing with pure, refined sugar . . . a substance which does not exist in nature and which never existed in any quantity in private homes until about the last 50 years or so. We are now eating an average of about 120 pounds of sugar a year—each of us.

We are using sugar in its most dangerous form (from the point of view of maintaining stable blood sugar levels)—that is, between meals, in coffee, candy and soft drinks, with no protein food to buffer the effects of this "drug"—for that's what it is.

Anyone "hooked" on sugar finds it easy to swing over to another addiction: black coffee, alcohol, cigarettes. All of them exert devastating effects on blood sugar levels. And from there it is only a step to stronger stuff, as long as nutritional health is neglected. We have more to say about hypoglycemia —or low blood sugar—later on in this book.

It is our firm belief that a nationwide program to supply high-protein meals, three or four or five a day, to people who are prone to addiction, along with megadoses of vitamins, could stop the addiction epidemic within a few years. It would be necessary to outlaw sugar or, at least, to label it as cigarettes are now labeled—"harmful to health" or perhaps "possibly leads to addiction."

Why has nothing of this kind ever been investigated? Why has no official health bureau ever studied the diet and the eating habits of addiction-prone individuals? The answer is in the letters we received from the health officials we queried about soft drinks. The general public has gotten used to eating this much sugar and "there is nothing harmful about it," so long as it does not edge out of the diet more nutritious foods, they tell us. How could it not? Doctors give coke to babies to help their digestion, although there is not a shred of scientific evidence that it ever does. But it's a lot easier and cheaper to keep the kids quiet with a dose of sugar than to investigate what is really wrong with them.

The food industry makes more money than any other industry, except the Pentagon. Cheap, sweet carbohydrates are the most profitable of all the products they make. Why should this industry give any research money to investigate whether such totally non-nutritious "foods" might be harming anyone?

These are only some of the many reasons why so many of us are addicted. They are also the reasons why the courageous men who are blazing a trail with orthomolecular psychiatry—megadoses of vitamins and high-protein diets—are having such a hard time gaining any official recognition. It's so much easier and strategic, as well as profitable, to look the other way and prate piously, "We really don't know what causes addiction." In a later chapter, we review a sensational new book, "Orthomolecular Psychiatry," edited by Dr. David Hawkins and Dr. Linus Pauling.

The *Lancet* reported in its January 6, 1973 issue on an individual physician who had been taking an addictive drug, and he found that large doses of folic acid, the B vitamin, decreased his withdrawal symptoms when he was unable to get a supply of this drug. He had been taking massive doses of the B vitamin (60 milligrams) daily for three years without any ill effects from the vitamin. The megadose approach is being used quite successfully in the treatment of alcoholism, drug addition and mental illness by Dr. David Hawkins and his colleagues at the North Nassau Mental Health Center, Long Island, New York. Dr. Hawkins is President of the Academy of Orthomolecular Psychiatry.

CHAPTER 9

Doctors Are Finding New Ways of Treating Schizophrenia

JOAN, THE 21-YEAR-OLD daughter of a business executive, began to display peculiar symptoms a month after she graduated from a fashionable college. She had hallucinations; she would repeat meaningless gestures over and over. The psychiatrists whom the family called in diagnosed schizophrenia and sent Joan to a mental hospital, where she was given the usual electric shock therapy and tranquilizers. Joan's story (her name has been disguised, of course) was told by Norman Cousins, editor of *Saturday Review*, in the December 10, 1972 issue of the *Philadelphia Inquirer*.

Joan grew steadily worse, finally becoming catatonic—that is, she would sit for long periods of time in a state of muscular rigidity, unable to relate to her surroundings. Her family, who could afford expensive doctors, called in consulting specialists.

Joan was shuttled from one hospital to another, and, over a five-year-period, she was in and out of seven medical centers. She had been exposed to many kinds of drugs and psychotherapy. Her parents paid bills amounting to $230,000, which wiped out their life savings and carried them heavily into debt.

Joan's brother and two sisters were distraught and suspicious all this time, because they thought that her illness might be hereditary and could affect them as well. In addition to the mental torment suffered by the family, there was serious disagreement over what kind of treatment Joan should have. The children thought one thing; the parents something else.

Finally, the tortured young woman was taken to a psychiatrist who believes that mental illness is a reflection of the physical condition of the body. He told Joan's family that she was suffering from pellagra—a disease involving deficiency in the B vitamin, niacin. During the depression of the 1930's, this disorder was almost as common as colds in the Southern United States, when poor people did not have enough niacin in their meals. But Joan's family was wealthy . . . how did it happen that she was suffering from pellagra?

It seems that Joan went on a crash diet one month before graduating from college. Her physician gave her amphetamines, the "pep" pill which supposedly cuts the appetite. Joan ate almost nothing and lost about 12 pounds a week. She found, too, that the pep pills could keep her going almost indefinitely without food, so she could stay awake all night

137

writing papers and cramming for exams.

In the space of a month, the strain on her nutritional reserves was so severe that she developed pellagra—but apparently only the mental symptoms of the deficiency disease. This is confirmation of the theory behind "orthomolecular psychiatry", which you will hear a great deal about in this book. This theory is that different parts of the body may be starving for nutrients while other areas show no deficiency symptoms. Joan had no skin or digestive symptoms. Her niacin deficiency involved only brain and nerve cells.

Said Norman Cousins: "Joan's pellagra and her schizoid symptoms have now disappeared as the result of a carefully supervised diet, fortified with heavy doses of ascorbic acid (vitamin C), niacin and other vitamins of the B Complex."

While Joan is slowly coming back to mental and physical health, she has a lot of natural doubts in her mind as to why her parents exposed her to these years of torment and why her case was not diagnosed correctly so many years ago. The parents, quite naturally, have many questions in their minds about why mental hospitals should be managed this way and why it has taken the general public and their physicians so long to learn that at least some kinds of mental illness have their basis in malnutrition.

This brings to mind a more tragic story. For about a week a young woman was observed living in Union Station in Washington, D.C. She was obviously penniless and had no place to live; her erratic behavior at times also showed that she was suffering

from some mental disorder. Railroad station police-
men were powerless to help her because of existing
District of Columbia laws. Finally, a newspaper
reporter, seeing her condition, bought her a few
meals and persuaded her to see a psychiatrist whom
he knew. She agreed to see the doctor, but, when
he suggested that she commit herself to a mental
hospital, she refused and asked to be taken "home"
to Union Station. During the interview, it was
learned that she had graduated from a well-known
college in the East, had worked for a time for a
famous New York magazine. She had ambitions to
become a successful writer, and, among her meager
possessions, were several books. A day or so later she
was found murdered in a dismal building near the
railroad station. In her impecunious condition, living
from hand to mouth for no telling how long, is there
any doubt that she was suffering from malnutrition,
which might have caused the mental aberrations?
Thus, she was easy prey for such a tragedy.

Schizophrenia, a form of mental illness, is a
major health hazard, afflicting at least two million
Americans, occurring most often among young men
and women from 16 to 30. It is estimated that three
out of every 100 people will be affected by schizophrenia during their lives. Babies born with the
disease are generally withdrawn, unhappy, moody
and excessively active. The disease may interfere
with speech and general learning development.
Many schizophrenic children are mistakenly diagnosed as mentally deficient.

Here are some of the symptoms to watch for:

1). Unaccountable changes in personality.

2). Perceptual changes—disturbances in seeing, hearing, touching, tasting and smelling—a distorted sense of time.

3). Hallucinations—strange visions and voices.

4). Disturbances in thought—delusions, suspicions, confusion, memory loss.

5). Extreme and prolonged depression, fatigue, apathy, fear, tension.

6). Bizarre behavior.

7). Headaches and insomnia.

8). In children: emotional disturbances, excessive activity, withdrawal, speech and learning difficulties.

Recently, a growing body of scientific evidence has shown that schizophrenia is the result of a defect in the body chemistry, probably inherited. Body chemicals carrying messages to the brain behave abnormally, causing the symptoms of schizophrenia.

A number of tests can be used to diagnose the disease. One of these (HOD test) and the EWI test measure the perceptual, thought and emotional disturbances of the patient. Physical tests can discover an abnormal substance in urine, disordered regulation of blood sugar levels and abnormal levels of histamine and trace minerals.

The "orthomolecular" approach provides for the individual person the optimum concentrations of important normal constituents of the brain. Psychiatrists, as we will see, who use this method may utilize any or all of the following in their treatment: several forms of niacin (B3), pyridoxine (B6), vitamin E, thyroid medication, vitamin B12, lithium (a trace mineral), vitamin C, plus several tranquilizers and anti-depressants. Where necessary, special diets aimed at correcting blood sugar levels are also used.

Early treatment, at the first sign of disorder, is most effective. The longer the disease progresses, the harder it may be to treat. An understanding family which will provide the patient with care and the means for following the prescribed treatment is essential.

Schizophrenia hospitalizes more patients than cancer, heart disease, and arthritis combined. More than half the total number of mental-hospital beds and one-fourth of all hospital beds in the U.S. are occupied by schizophrenics. The *average* stay of a schizophrenia patient in a mental hospital is estimated at 15 years.

Our nation loses $1 billion a year in earning power, $200 million in federal taxes, and spends $350 million for care and treatment of schizophrenics. Including the cost of private care for non-hospitalized patients, the cost of this disorder comes to $2 billion annually. The real cost is human wreckage—unemployment, poverty, broken homes, degradation, suicide.

"Without effective treatment, schizophrenics are condemned to a twilight existence between life and death, many spending their lives in mental institutions, others within reach of their families but unreachable. . . . We must make every effort to halt the relentless drain on human and financial resources caused by schizophrenia. As citizens and taxpayers, we must demand a new emphasis upon expanded research efforts and the application of effective diagnostic and treatment methods."

These words are from a booklet, "What You Can Do About Schizophrenia," which is available from the American Schizophrenia Association, 56 West 45th Street, New York City 10036. If you know of someone who has a family problem with this disorder, ask them to get in touch with the Association for help and direction to a doctor who uses this method of treatment, and/or a local group of interested citizens who are supporting the work of this Association in various parts of the United States. At the end of this book, we list names and addresses of some of the doctors, clinics, etc.

Dr. Russell Smith of Michigan, describing his experience with alcoholics, tells us that benefits from treatment with massive doses of niacin may appear within a few weeks or it may take several years. Three out of four persons treated derive benefit from niacin therapy and show dramatic changes in their ability to abstain from drinking. Many of the same effects seen in alcoholics taking the niacin treatment are also seen in adolescents with acute or chronic brain damage, especially damage caused by drug abuse or the use of hallucinatory drugs like LSD.

Furthermore, those who derive no benefit or little benefit from the vitamin therapy (approximately one out of every four patients) usually discontinue its use, so little time or effort is wasted in vain attempts to cure. On the other hand, when a successful therapy is interrupted, changes in the patient are so undesirable that he quickly resumes therapy of his own volition.

What are some of the benefits gained and the reason for failure? Dr. Smith says that failure in some cases may be the result of simple lack of knowledge as to how best to use the vitamin and measure its effects. This is a new therapy, comparatively speaking. Doctors have been treating mental illness and alcoholism for thousands of years. Only within the past 20 years or so has anyone experimented with megavitamin therapy—that is, therapy which uses extremely large (mega) doses of certain vitamins.

Some of the benefits noted in patients successfully treated are these: improved sleep patterns, reduced anxiety, stabilized moods (in other words, fewer abrupt swings from depression to excitement), increased ability to solve problems, absence of "dry drunks," reduced alcohol tolerance and reduced severity of withdrawal. Patients also report occasional dramatic improvement in judgment and memory, protection against heart attacks and strokes, sustained better performance on the job, improved family life and better integration into Alcoholics Anonymous. It is noteworthy that the doctors working with this series of patients are great believers in A.A. Their patients attend meetings regularly.

Dr. Smith's report also mentions that large doses of the B vitamin niacin also reduce blood cholesterol and, in general, produce a lowering of blood pressure. In the same leaflet which carries Dr. Smith's article appears a letter from Dr. Edwin Boyle, Jr. of the Miami Heart Institute who said: "Niacin is one of the most promising drugs currently available to lower blood fats and cholesterol and help reduce death and disability from heart attacks. Heart attacks kill more alcoholics than any other cause. This unusual vitamin tends to 'normalize' blood clotting and blood fats as well as help overcome certain nervous disorders."

Dr. Boyle goes on to say that the federal government is presently sponsoring a study known as the National Coronary Drug Project under a branch of the National Institutes of Health. The American Heart Association and the FDA are cooperating. Four drugs are being tested for their effectiveness in preventing heart attacks. One of the "drugs" is niacin. It was chosen because of its ability to lower blood cholesterol and blood fat.

The Safety Monitoring Committee of this project, after three years of using niacin, has pronounced it safe for humans, even in doses as high as 3,000 milligrams daily. Dr. Boyle uses it in doses up to 4,000 milligrams and says his results are "most encouraging." The recommended dietary allowances for niacin are: infants (5 to 8 mg. daily); children (8 to 15 mg. daily); males (17 to 20 mg. daily); females (13 to 15 mg. daily); pregnant women (15 mg. daily); lactating women (20 mg. daily); to give you an idea of what enormous doses are being used successfully in megavitamin therapy.

Dr. Smith believes that these large doses of niacin may act more like a hormone than a vitamin. A hormone is a substance produced by a body gland for some role in body metabolism. Dr. Smith is convinced that one of the most important parts of the niacin therapy for alcoholics is that it "seems to make a significant difference in the ability to obtain and maintain alcohol abstinence." Until now, no biological weapon has been available to help the alcoholic control his craving for alcohol. True, there are "negative" controls, such as Antabuse, which will make the victim ill if he drinks. But this is a negative approach. How much more advantageous is a simple, harmless vitamin which prevents the craving for booze.

At his Manhasset, New York clinic, Dr. David Hawkins has an astonishing track record in using megavitamin therapy to deal with schizophrenia and alcoholism. The clinic has treated over 4,000 patients, about 600 of whom were alcoholics. "The great majority of this large group have exhibited very marked improvement. Most of them could be called recovered, if we define 'recovery' as the ability to function satisfactorily in the community with little or no professional help," Dr. Hawkins stated.

Dr. Hawkins notes that there is a vast difference in time and expense involved with megavitamin therapy. At most mental health clinics, there are extensive interviews with psychiatric personnel, a process which may involve months and which produces only a diagnosis, no treatment.

Using the megavitamin therapy, doctors at the New York clinic may see the patient only 15 times the first year, four to six times the second year. These are "severely ill people, many of them having multiple problems, as well as schizophrenia." Tests to determine the patient's condition are quickly done, since they are largely biochemical tests.

A study published by the American Schizophrenia Association in 1971 showed that treatment of patients by the "new" orthomolecular methods slashed costs to the patient by 90 per cent. Using rapid screening tests, large doses of selected vitamins, plus high-protein, low-carbohydrate diets and a certain amount of tranquilizers, anti-depressants and psychotherapy, Dr. Hawkins showed that his clinic could treat seriously ill schizophrenics for $200 per patient and reduce the average number of patient visits to the office from 150 per year to 15.

In a preface to the report, Senator Harold Hughes of Iowa stated: "Dr. Hawkins' report should have the attention of responsible medical and public officials. Dr. Hawkins described a treatment system designed to enable millions of Americans afflicted with schizophrenia, and their families, to live more satisfying lives without bankrupting themselves in the process. I believe that mental health program administrators at every level owe it to their patients and their communities to investigate Dr. Hawkins' system and give it proper trial."

Dr. Abram Hoffer, President of the Huxley Institute for Biosocial Research and the American Schizophrenia Association, said: "It is our feeling that such a study could have tremendous impact on the quality and availability of treatment for schizophrenia. The possibilities for reducing the staggering costs of schizophrenia to the patient and the taxpayer, and providing effective treatment to many more than now receive it, are worthy of the highest priority."

There are three circumstances which complicate the patient's recovery at Dr. Hawkins' clinic; three problems which appear over and over again. First, patients may be taking drugs—hypnotics or barbiturates (sleeping pills or tranquilizers). "In every single case where these medications have been used, the effect was noticeably deleterious," Dr. Hawkins remarked.

Second, many patients were suffering from low blood sugar, which had gone undetected by doctors they had previously seen. "Such alcoholic patients immediately felt better as soon as they were taken off sugar and sweets and placed on (niacin) to elevate their blood sugar levels."

Those alcoholics who took six-hour glucose tolerance tests for low blood sugar reported that, during the test, they experienced many of the feelings which they had felt so often and which led them to drinking as the only possible remedy.

"Quite a few patients who had been sober for considerable lengths of time reported periodic depression, feelings of tension, anxiety and recurrent desires to drink. By correcting the low blood sugar, they could eliminate these symptoms."

The third problem in some of the alcoholic patients is the presence of many distortions in perceptions such as schizophrenics experience: taste, hearing, seeing, perception of one's own body parts, the sense of time and space are disordered in ways that make the patient do and say peculiar things. Yet it is almost impossible for him to explain to well people what is causing his strangeness.

In some patients, says the report, it was difficult to know if it was a case of schizophrenia complicated by alcoholism, or a case of alcoholism complicated by schizophrenia. When such patients do not improve under treatment, the report suggests the reason may be permanent brain damage on a biochemical basis—because of the body's misuse of adrenalin, a hormone of the adrenal glands, which is involved in the body's reaction to stress.

Here, briefly, are some astonishing case histories of patients treated at the New York clinic:

1). A 33-year-old housewife who had been severely ill with schizophrenia for five years. She had been treated by a number of highly qualified psychiatrists. She had had many drugs in massive doses and electroshock treatment.

Her doctor finally recommended a prefrontal lobotomy—an operation to destroy a part of the brain. Her psychiatrist became furious when megavitamin therapy was suggested, and refused to consider it. The patient was also convinced the therapy would not help, but she consented to try it. She was given megavitamins, thyroid gland medication, the diet to correct low blood sugar (see a later chapter for such a diet) and a small dose of tranquilizers. In 10 weeks she recovered, returned home and has been well since then.

2). A 45-year-old man was diagnosed as a "chronic paranoid schiozphrenic" for 10 years. He had lengthy hospitalization, all the available drugs, shock treatment and insulin coma therapy. His condition was "deplorable." He screamed obscenities at his imagined enemies, could not speak a coherent sentence, refused to take any medication and ate sporadically a "bizarre" choice of foods.

Since he refused to take pills, a mixture of vitamin C and niacin was given him in his coffee, disguised so that he would not detect it. (He was a big coffee drinker). By the end of a year he had improved to such an extent that he was calm, had no hallucinations, read the paper, looked for a job and is still unaware that he is getting the megavitamin therapy.

3). A 23-year-old man had been schizophrenic since childhood and had become involved with almost every drug the drug addict knows. When he was finally picked up on the street by the police, who brought him to Bellevue Hospital, he was injecting $140 worth of methedrine every day and suffering from needle hepatitis.

On the megavitamin therapy his hallucinations disappeared, along with the craving for drugs. He is now "moving on to a responsible job involving administrative responsibility in the counseling of young people who are still quite ill due to drugs plus schizophrenia."

4). A 28-year-old man had been ill for six years. He was brought to the hospital in a pitiful condition of starvation, for he had decided to refuse food and thus commit suicide, so despondent was he over his own mental condition. He had "spent the last four years at one of the highest priced, famous psychoanalytically oriented, private psychiatric hospitals in the United States."

His therapy to that point had cost almost $200,000 and had reduced him to this terrible condition. On the megavitamin therapy and some mild tranquilizers, he was discharged within 10 weeks, is now leading an active social life and has a good job.

In addition to the high-protein diet given patients in the megavitamin therapy, what vitamins do they take? Niacin is given in doses of four grams (4,000 milligrams) daily. Vitamin C is given in doses of four grams daily. Fifty milligrams of vitamin B6 (pyridoxine) are also given daily. In many cases, vitamin E was given in doses of 200 units four times a day.

These are truly massive doses and they are, apparently, entirely harmless. No ill effects are reported in any of these cases. This is in sharp contrast to many ill effects often produced by psychiatric drugs and the many accidents that can occur with insulin shock and electroshock therapy.

Credit is given throughout Dr. Smith's article and Dr. Hawkins' article to Dr. Humphrey Osmond, Dr. Abram Hoffer and Professor Linus Pauling, who are pioneers in the field of orthomolecular psychiatry.

We believe that this successful therapy has potential for uncovering much that is wrong in current thinking about nutrition and nutritional supplements. We also think that this is one of the most important developments in the long, long history of mental illness, drug addiction and alcoholism which have blighted so many lives. Says Dr. Smith: "We must solicit financial support, advice, criticism, interest and direction through the usual channels of scientific communication, governmental regulatory agencies and the scientific community at large."

Unfortunately, however, this is like running into a brick wall. It is our experience in the health food field that interest and support for any simple, inexpensive treatment, utilizing chiefly diet supplements, never develops until the general public demands that it be forthcoming. If this book can somehow move more people in that direction, then our efforts have not been in vain.

In a 1970 issue of *Psychosomatics* 11(5), pages 517-521, Dr. D. R. Hawkins, A. W. Bortin and R. P. Runyon report on 80 schizophrenic patients who were given megadoses of vitamin B. They had a relapse rate half that of a control group of 80 patients who did not receive the vitamin therapy.

Dr. Abram Hoffer in *Schizophrenia*, 2 (2-3), pages 80-86, 1970, describes the case of a psychiatrist who suffered from the rapid onset of schizophrenia at the age of 56. He developed distressing symptoms of disorganization in the way he saw, felt and smelled things, his thoughts were disordered, he had acute depression, great bewilderment and vague but terrible fears. He suffered from visual hallucinations —the same general type that occurs with overdoses of some hallucinogenic drugs like LSD. Apparently these symptoms had been bothering the physician for more than 10 years, but neither he nor his relatives had recognized them as symptoms of schizophrenia. More than 40 years earlier he had experimented with the hallucinogenic drug mescaline, and the symptoms he now felt were much like those induced by that drug. In spite of the long time that his symptoms had been with him, he responded very rapidly to massive doses of nicotinic acid and vitamin C, along with a sugar-free diet.

In *Schizophrenia*, volume 2 (4), pages 177-179, 1970, Dr. Allan Cott, a New York specialist who utilizes megadoses of vitamins, reviews the use of injections of large doses of B vitamins and vitamin C, along with large doses by mouth. He said that clinical response was generally seen by the end of the second week of treatment. These were patients who had achieved some improvement by taking vitamins orally. In a second group, hospitalized because of the severity of their illness, there was a more rapid response than in the patients who did not have injections. The vitamins (vitamin B3, or niacin; vitamin C; vitamin B1, or thiamine; and vitamin B6, or pyridoxine) were injected intramuscularly three times a week. Oral doses of the same vitamins in large amounts were continued at the same time.

"I think schizophrenia is a disease where there is relative deficiency of vitamin B3," said Dr. Abram Hoffer in November 1971, speaking at a joint conference of the Canadian and American Schizophrenia Associations and the Schizophrenia Association of Great Britain. "Certain people require more than is provided in the diet. If we were to add at least one gram (1,000 milligrams) a day, we could, in the next decade or two, see a very significant decrease in the extent of this disease."

Dr. Hoffer stated that he has 2,000 case records of schizophrenia patients treated with massive doses of vitamins. Patients were given, first, three grams of niacin, plus one gram of vitamin C a day. If the patients were very anxious, they also got tranquilizers and anti-depressants. "A nutritional survey was also made," Dr. Hoffer continued, "since we find many people do not eat properly." If the patient improved in the first month, the treatment was continued until he was completely free from symptoms. If he did not respond, he was hospitalized and given other regular psychiatric treatment, along with increased doses of vitamins.

One patient needed 30 grams (30,000 milligrams) of niacin daily to stay in good health. If the dosage dropped to 24 grams, her symptoms returned. In part three of the treatment, the administration of megadoses of vitamins may continue for up to seven years. And Dr. Hoffer claims a more than 90 per cent recovery rate with schizophrenics who have been ill for one year or less. The remaining 10 per cent become better, though not well. Those who had been chronically ill for up to 20 years, but continue to live in the community, showed a 75 per cent recovery rate. With patients who had been in mental hospitals, Dr. Hoffer was lucky to get 10 per cent recovery.

In *Schizophrenia* 3(1), pages 41-46, 1971, Dr. Hoffer describes an entire family dependent on large doses of vitamin B for good health. The father had been given nicotinic acid (a form of niacin) for treatment of an eye condition and he was later hospitalized as a schizophrenic. He was given a daily maintenance dose of nicotinic acid, which controlled his symptoms. His oldest son, an alcoholic, was also found to be schizophrenic; his two sisters were also schizophrenic. He and they were able to control their illness with large doses of nicotinic acid. Patients often ask whether mental illness and/or alcoholism are inherited. This story seems to indicate that the *susceptibility* to both may be inherited. Whether or not one succumbs to either disease may be related in some way to the kind of life one lives. Perhaps a well-nourished individual, getting large amounts of vitamins and minerals daily, and observing other rules of good health—such as ample sleep and exercise—may be able to withstand the onset of these pernicious diseases, even though he has inherited the susceptibility. Why not? And why isn't somebody doing world-wide experiments to see if such a theory is correct?

Two California physicians, who have been treating a variety of conditions with vitamin E, have a letter to the editor in *Lancet* (July 15, 1972). They discuss a previous *Lancet* article in which a doctor reported giving "high doses" of vitamin E to two patients with the serious mental illness of manic depressive psychosis. The doctor had found these "high doses" to be ineffective.

Said Drs. Samuel Ayers and Richard Mihan: "Where vitamin E is indicated in therapeutic amounts, an effective dose would be certainly not less than 400 I.U. (International Units, roughly equivalent to milligrams) daily and, more likely, 800 to 1,600 I.U. daily." They go on to tell of excellent results in treating some "intractable" skin conditions as well as night cramps in the legs and "restless legs." They happened to discover the effectiveness of vitamin E for the leg conditions when they gave it for the skin conditions.

"Vitamin E may or may not be effective in the control of manic-depressive psychoses, but it certainly seems to be unwise to conclude that it was ineffective on the basis of a grossly inadequate dose and in a trial on only two people," the doctors added.

Dr. George Prastka of the Capistrano-by-the-Sea Neuropsychiatric Hospital, Dana Point, Calif., says that he has found in the early stages of schizophrenia that about 50 per cent of patients will respond favorably to large doses of vitamin B3 and vitamin C, and that other vitamins of the B Complex are also used as supplements. Dr. Prastka was addressing the Orange County chapter of the American Schizophrenia Association, and his remarks were reported in the *Fullerton Daily News Tribune.*

Admitting that the use of megadoses of vitamins is still a controversial issue, Dr. Prastka said that "the people who have been the most critical seem to me to have been those who have not tried it." He indicated however, that megavitamins are becoming more acceptable, especially in the eastern United States and in Europe, and he mentioned the National Institutes of Health 4-year-study that we discussed earlier. He was critical of the use of anti-depressants, which he said can produce disabling side effects.

"About half of all hospital beds are occupied by

patients with emotional disease and about half of them have been diagnosed as schizophrenic," Dr. Prastka said. "It is a disease manifested primarily by symptoms exhibiting a pronounced separation between a person's logical mind and his feelings."

Mental disorders are commonly associated with disability and long-stay hospitalization, as Dr. Prastka has indicated. This was corroborated by *Statistical Bulletin* for December 1972. Death rates among those suffering from such disorders are higher than those experienced in the general population. The magnitude of the problem of mental disorders is highlighted by a study the National Center for Health Statistics made during April-June 1963 of adult patients, ages 15 and over in 414 long-stay mental hospitals in the United States. There were about 560,000 patients in these hospitals, not counting those under maximum security, in children's wards, and in mental hospitals serving children only.

The length of stay was determined as the time elapsing between the patient's last admission to the hospital and the day the survey was taken. It does not necessarily represent the total time the individual has been in mental hospitals. In 1963, the average stay in a mental hospital was 6½ years. The shortest stay was for patients under 45 years of age (about three years), but, as the age goes up, the length of stay increases to 10 years for patients 55 to 64 years old. About two-fifths of the patients in all hospitals surveyed had been there for 10 years or longer.

Neuroses, personality disorders and other non-psychotic mental disorders killed almost 5,000 people in 1968—equivalent to 2.5 people in every 100,000 . . . 3,900 of these were alcoholics. A study of mortality in New York State mental institutions showed that, in both sexes, the death rates for the institutionalized were seven times those for the general population.

Here is a letter from a Connecticut psychiatrist which appeared in *Schizophrenia Bulletin,* published by the National Institute of Mental Health, in Washington, a federal government bureau.

"I am a board-certified psychiatrist with a large private practice and a large experience with drug therapy in schizophrenia. I have used nicotinic acid (vitamin B3) for at least two or three years, with other vitamins, in treatment of schizophrenia—sometimes routinely and sometimes only when the regular phenothiazine medication would not clear the symptoms completely. In about 80 per cent of my cases there was an improvement when I introduced large doses of nicotinic acid with vitamin C, especially in areas of perception and ability to concentrate. It is interesting that patients themselves felt a great relief after started on this medication and urged me to continue.

"Side effects were few and rare, because I advised my patients to take a glass of cold milk or an antihistamine together with nicotinic acid and told them to always take it after meals. The maximum dosage I have used is three grams (3,000 milligrams) a day of nicotinic acid and the same amount of vitamin C. I insist that, if taken correctly and according to the above-mentioned advice, side effects are very rare.

157

Even though there is no really logical and comprehensive explanation of the mode of action of megavitamin therapy, the fact remains that it is successful as an empirical treatment. In my case, I use it only as an addition to psychotherapy and phenothiazines (tranquilizers)."

Symptoms of schizophrenia may be produced by a normal protein, which goes out of control because of a reduction in its regulating enzyme system, according to a team of Detroit investigators who reported at a meeting of the American Psychiatric Association in 1972. They believe that certain abnormal substances may thus be produced in certain sections of the brain, which could be responsible for the schizophrenic symptoms.

"The probability is great that there are other metabolites, as yet unidentified, and other areas of the brain involved," they said, as reported in *Medical Tribune* for June 14, 1972.

Dr. Bella Kowalson, a general practitioner in Winnipeg, Canada, spoke on diet and its relation to mental health at a meeting of the Canadian Schizophrenia Foundation in 1970. She pointed out that the brain is a part of the body and the mind is one of its functions. So when we say, "We are what we eat," we are in essence saying that our brains too are what we eat, since they have nothing on which to build good health except for the food and water we provide in our diets.

Malnutrition may result from any of a number of "slips twixt the cup and the lip," in the way of improper choice of foods, inefficient digestion, inefficient absorption and improper utilization of food in the various chemical processes that take place in human cells. Malnutrition may result from a deficiency in any of these processes or a failure to compensate for increased requirements for various nutrients.

For example, pernicious anemia used to be a fatal disease, always. No one understood what caused it. Now we know that it is caused by lack of vitamin B12 in the diet, or by lack of the individual's ability to absorb vitamin B12 in meals. The deficiency disease pellagra which has mental symptoms very much like those of schizophrenia comes about from lack of an amino acid or form of protein, plus lack of a B vitamin, niacin. "Pellagra has been considered by some authorities to be one of the most serious deficiency diseases in the United States," said Dr. Kowalson.

She goes on to point out that man, in his misguided attempts to make foods more palatable and profitable, discards or loses many of the nutrients which are essential to health—mental health as well as physical. Refining cereals and the flour from which bread is made causes disastrous loss of B vitamins. Improper cooking methods destroy the B complex, vitamin C and many minerals.

"The refinement and concentration of natural carbohydrates has presented them for human consumption in quantities which our bodies were never meant to handle. The increased intake of refined sugars tends to overstimulate the pancreatic gland, resulting in overproduction of insulin. This in turn results in a fall in the normal level of blood glucose (sugar)," Dr. Kowalson said. The brain depends on blood sugar, almost entirely, for proper functioning. So when this supply is cut off, as in conditions of hypoglycemia or low blood sugar, the brain cannot function properly.

As we will discover later in the chapter on hypoglycemia, this influx of insulin primes the adrenal glands to produce an overabundance of its hormones —a situation which also prevails when the body is under special stress. This overstimulation produces symptoms of anxiety, nervousness, dizziness, sweating and so on. Over a period of time, this depresses many body functions and creates abnormal fatigue. Vitamin C, which is abundant in the adrenal glands, is also used up rapidly, creating a deficiency which cannot be alleviated with the very small amount of this vitamin in the average daily diet.

"As some of you may know," Dr. Kowalson went on, "I am dissatisfied with the current unscientific and emotionally charged misnomer of schizophrenia. This label adds to the burden of shame, guilt, inadequacy and despair of those afflicted with it. I have suggested that the name 'metabolic dysperception' be used to describe this illness which is characterized by dysfunction of sensory perception, with corresponding changes in thought, mood and behavior. The fact that it responds favorably to megavitamin B3 and allied therapy proves it is of metabolic or biochemical origin."

The Canadian Schizophrenia Foundation has pamphlets available on this subject. Write to them and ask what they have. Their address is: 200 A Brent Building, 2505 Eleventh Ave., Regina, Saskatchewan, Canada.

A New Zealand doctor, Dr. Michael H. Briggs, has been using vitamin C in the treatment of schizophrenia. He said, in the *British Medical Journal,* that patients in mental hospitals may suffer from chronic lack of vitamin C because of poor dietary habits. They simply cannot be made to eat enough of the fresh raw foods which are our most dependable source of this illusive vitamin.

But, said Dr. Briggs, there is another reason why schizophrenics may be short on vitamin C. It has been found, he said, that these mental patients may have an overabundance of copper in their blood. One investigator has shown that the amounts of copper in the blood fluctuate rapidly in emotional states. So when mental patients become agitated, as they may several times a day, the copper content of their blood may increase rapidly. We do not know how or why this should be, but we do know that copper is very destructive of vitamin C. It burns up vitamin C, or ascorbic acid, whenever it comes into contact with it. So, it would seem that these disturbed people may lose large amounts of vitamin C each time they have an emotional upset.

Dr. Briggs reports that chronic schizophrenics excrete considerably more vitamin C than other types of mental patients. This, too, would seem to indicate that the copper blood level brought about by their excitement is causing them to lose vitamin C.

The New Zealand investigator believes that being constantly short on vitamin C could lead to an imbalance of other substances in the liver which might allow some unwanted substance to accumulate, leading to mental disturbance. Thus, lack of vitamin C could lead to a disturbed mental condition, which might cause high levels of copper in the blood, which would destroy even more vitamin C, thus setting up a cycle that would condemn the patient to chronic mental illness. As we have reported through this book, many researchers utilize vitamin C and the B vitamins quite successfully.

While we are on the subject of vitamin C, we will discuss a new book by Albert Szent-Györgyi, one of the most distinguished biologists alive and the discoverer of this vitamin. It is called *The Living State, With Observations on Cancer*. It is not for the layman; it was written for other biologists and chemists. But it contains a number of things of a startling nature. One of the most interesting is how he discovered that wheat germ and vitamin C keep him from having colds. This is what Dr. Szent-Györgyi has for breakfast: a sliced banana, over which he pours about two ounces of wheat germ (about half a cup). Then he adds milk, as you do for any breakfast cereal. Then he has a cup of tea to which he has added vitamin C in a mixture with sugar, which makes the vitamin less tart. The heaping spoonful of this mixture contains about one gram (1,000 milligrams) of vitamin C. In the afternoon he takes another cup of tea with the same amount of vitamin C.

If you want to follow this general plan to see if it will protect you, too, against colds, it would be wise to take the vitamin C along with your morning wheat germ, no matter in what form the vitamin may be: pills, powder, liquid, etc. And do take enough of it, although we would suggest that you try to avoid the sugar. Dr. Szent-Györgyi feels very strongly, as Dr. Linus Pauling does, that the effectiveness of vitamin C in preventing colds is closely related to the amount you take. If you are not taking enough to satisfy your own individual needs, you may not be successful.

"I have always felt," said Dr. Szent-Györgyi, "that not enough use was made of ascorbic acid. Those who say that if one does not have scurvy he is getting plenty of vitamin C are wrong, for scurvy is not the first symptom of lack of vitamin C. It is a sign of the final collapse of the organism, a premortal syndrome, and there is a very wide gap between scurvy and a completely healthy condition. Good health is a state in which we feel best, work best, and have the greatest resistance to disease. Nobody knows how far we are from such a state."

If you get pneumonia, the doctor's diagnosis will be pneumonia, not malnutrition, even though it may have been a state of malnutrition which causes you to be susceptible to the pneumonia. The doctor has probably treated you only for pneumonia—not malnutrition.

But why should our bodies be so frail that they should be forever breaking down before the onslaught of a cold or some other kind of disorder? Said Dr. Szent-Györgyi: "I am often shocked at the eating habits of people. What I find difficult to understand as a biologist is not why people become ill, but how they manage to stay alive at all. Our body must be a very wonderful instrument to with-. stand all our insults."

Dr. Szent-Györgyi then relates several stories of how Europeans were cured of various disorders when they were given massive doses of vitamin C. One of these was a mentally ill person who had taken incredibly large amounts and had come to no harm. "Vitamin C is harmless," he continues. "It does not injure your health nor your pocketbook, being a very cheap commodity."

Dr. Szent-Györgyi tells us he knows of one boy who was "completely antisocial." He was given vitamin C and became congenial. The arguments against using large amounts of vitamin C are not sound, he says. True, you may excrete some vitamin C in your urine, if you take more than you need. So what?

CHAPTER 10

Vitamin Therapy for Hyperactive "Problem" Children

EVIDENCE IS ACCUMULATING daily that many forms of mental disorder, from schizophrenia to hyperactivity in children, can be treated successfully with diet and massive doses of certain vitamins. Dr. Abram Hoffer is one of the many psychiatrists who are using this method of treatment. The *Canadian Medical Journal* for July 22, 1972 contains a letter to the editor from Dr. Hoffer describing yet another case in his practice where the improvement of a hyperactive, hyperkinetic, "problem" child was unbelievably rapid, when he was given massive doses of only two B vitamins.

Said Dr. Hoffer: "I would like to present one case in order to illustrate the kind of results which might be expected. This young patient, aged 14, was first seen April 6, 1972. The chairman of the Pupil Services Department of the Board of Education stated that for the first three months of 1972 the patient did not work at school, was disruptive a good deal of the time, came to school late and left without permission, and engaged in bizarre behavior, such as smearing blood all over his face from a small cut on his hand. He was not bad all the time but had many bad days and when he was bad he was apparently horrid.

"His behavior became so strange and bizarre that it was impossible to leave him alone," Dr. Hoffer continues. "His actions were summarized as being very impulsive and completely unpredictable, and he seemed never to learn anything. It was the conclusion of the teacher that there was something seriously wrong with this patient and that they could no longer deal with him at school. His I.Q. was around 80 but this was obviously much too low, because he seemed to be of normal intelligence.

"The patient's mother reported that he had been somewhat hyperactive most of his life but that he had become much worse over the past two years," Dr. Hoffer said. "He was referred to a child psychiatrist who, after several examinations, reported that he was normal and that he would grow out of his problem. However, he did not and he continued to present very difficult problems at school and began to develop behavior problems at home."

Dr. Hoffer goes on to describe some of the imaginary things bothering the boy, which he uncovered by giving him an examination designed to bring out this kind of disturbance. The boy thought that people were "watching" him. He saw faces in the air. He heard his name being called when no one was calling him. He felt that he could hear his own thinking inside his head. He was sure that people were making fun of him and running him down, gossiping about him.

In addition, he was extremely restless, irritable and cranky, and so hyperactive that on this score he stood within the range of schizophrenia. Dr. Hoffer gave the child two B vitamins—niacinamide and pyridoxine—three grams of the former per day, and ½ gram of the latter. These are massive doses. The official recommendation for a daily diet level of niacin is 20 milligrams for a boy this age. Dr. Hoffer prescribed almost 3,000 times that amount. The daily recommendation for vitamin B6 is 2 milligrams. Dr. Hoffer prescribed 250 times this much.

The child was to report back one month later. He cancelled the appointment because he was working, selling ice cream. At the end of May he came to the doctor's office, reported that he felt better, was getting good grades in school, had no trouble getting along with the other children. He had received an excellent report from the teacher who had considered him as almost hopeless before this. His mother and the teacher corroborated this testimony. The boy was completely re-made.

Could the results have been due to some psychological reaction to Dr. Hoffer? He says this is quite impossible. The child had seen psychiatrists on several occasions before with no results and his session with Dr. Hoffer was no more than one-half hour long.

Dr. Hoffer concludes his letter with this proposal,

very modest considering the sensational quality of the successful treatment he has just described. He says, "Since it is a general scientific rule that where one patient will respond to particular treatment there must be others who will also do so, I suggest that all physicians try treating hyperkinetic children with these vitamins which seem to be so effective in my hands."

Speaking before the Senate Select Committee on Nutrition and Human Needs, March 2, 1971, Dr. Charles C. Edwards, then Commissioner, Food and Drug Administration, had this to say:

"Of considerable interest (to the FDA) are the findings in a series of research projects concerned with the relationship of nutrition to the mental and physical development of children. There are more than 25 specific research projects in this area that are funded at the level of $2.7 million. They deal with such diverse aspects of the subject as the effect of malnutrition in pregnancy on the number of brain cells in the newborn infant to the critical study of social development after malnutrition in infancy.

"The reversible, but serious, effects on learning of moderately severe undernutrition are being documented. As many as 30 per cent to 40 per cent of some primary school population in this country may be involved with these nutritionally related learning handicaps," Dr. Edwards said.

These alarming statistics brought to mind two press releases that we received some time ago. One of the releases stated, "The outcome of a nutritional survey of over 600 children from New York City's lower East Side indicates that not all American children are well nourished.

Poor diets, low vitamin levels and below average size and weight were found in certain groups of children in an analysis by New Jersey College of Medicine and Dentistry physicians, a New York physician and a statistician. In one group of Puerto Rican children low levels of vitamin C, vitamin B3 and vitamin B12 were found. These same children had low reading levels, a finding which points to the need for good nutrition in order to perform well in school. This was in contrast with a group of Chinese children who showed very high reading scores. These youngsters were on good diets and had high levels of vitamin B1 and vitamin B6. In the Chinese group, however, 30 per cent took supplementary vitamins.

A striking feature of another group of children was very low vitamin B2 levels. "The importance of riboflavin deficiency as a general nutritional problem has been emphasized", the investigators noted. These children were also low in all B vitamins except folic acid and vitamin B1, as well as vitamin C.

In one group low levels of vitamin B2 and vitamins B6 and B12 were discovered. Most of these children came from families in which the mother was the main wage earner. "The mother's absence during the day may explain the frequent finding of a poor dietary history," according to the scientists. "Maternal neglect or rejection has been shown to be correlated with decreased height, weight and bone maturation."

The other press release, from the Metropolitan Life Insurance Company, stated: "In 1966, about 3,629,000 babies were born in the United States and about 84,800 died in their first year of life." These figures translate into a rate of 23.4 infant deaths per 1,000 live births, a figure that suggests plenty of room for improvement. Consequently, the United States is 15th among all nations in figures on infant mortality. The following countries lose fewer babies than we do: Scotland, France, Israel, Japan, Czechoslovakia, England and Wales, Switzerland, Australia, Denmark, New Zealand, Finland, Norway, Netherlands and Sweden.

Could not these figures be the outcome of conditions of wretchedly poor nutrition—from the fetus to the grave—among whole groups of people in our country? Is it any wonder that we have so many hyperactive children and those with learning disabilities?

Dr. Allan Cott, a private psychiatrist who practices in New York, is another specialist who believes in the megavitamin approach for these troubled children. In an article, "Orthomolecular Approach to the Treatment of Learning Disabilities," in *Schizophrenia*, Volume 3, Number 2, Dr. Cott tells us that, in the last five years, he has treated 500 children with large doses of vitamins and has had better results than he has had with any other kind of treatment. He says there are very few cases of dramatic response by disturbed children treated with the usual drugs. In an earlier chapter we mentioned that some schools are using drugs to treat "difficult" or hyperactive children. Dr. Cott tells us that the response of the children to these drugs is poor.

Dr. Cott has successfully treated adults with massive doses of niacin, vitamin B6, vitamin C, vitamin E and others, especially those patients with schizophrenia. So he began treatment of schizophrenic and autistic (daydreamers) children and "found improvement in many of these children to be more dramatic than in adults." He said that the treatment is most effective if it is given to difficult children when they are quite young. As they grow older, longer and longer treatment is needed.

His descriptions of these unfortunate children are arresting. He indicates that, in most instances, within three to six months the child begins to understand and obey commands. He shows a willingness to cooperate with parents and teachers. The hyperactivity which is one of the main symptoms of the childhood mental troubles—begins to subside.

The children who are brought to him have been exposed to "every form of treatment and every known tranquilizer and sedative with little or no success, even in controlling the hyperactivity." After treatment with massive vitamin therapy, those who have never spoken begin to babble. Those who can already speak begin to show steady improvement in forming phrases and short sentences. "In their general behavior, they show a greater appreciation for the people in their environment. They become more loving and not only permit cuddling and hugging, but seek it. Bizarre food choices change slowly to include a larger variety of foods," Dr. Cott added.

Dr. Cott gives disturbed children and children with learning disabilities these vitamins: niacin or niacinamide—one to two grams daily depending on body weight; vitamin C—one to two grams daily; vitamin B6—200 to 400 milligrams daily; and calcium pantothenate (this is one form of the B vitamin pantothenic acid)—400 to 600 milligrams daily. These are starting doses for little ones weighing 35 pounds or more, he said. He varies the dose depending on individual response.

He adds that, in the Soviet Union, doctors are also using vitamin B15 (pangamic acid) in cases of retardation. They believe it helps supply oxygen to brain tissues. This vitamin is not officially listed as being a vitamin in any literature in the United States.

In his article, Dr. Cott discusses a brain-injured child who had had seizures every day for three years. Eleven days after he started on vitamin B6 therapy, he had his first day free from these attacks. During all those years he had been taking the tranquilizers usually prescribed for this condition and the seizures had not stopped.

Another child who had multiple daily seizures for two years became free from seizures 72 hours after the massive doses of vitamins were begun. He was still well four years later. "I have seen very few cases of childhood schizophrenia, autism or brain injury in whom seizure activity did not respond to the megavitamins," Dr. Cott said.

Parents bringing their children for this treatment and watching their steady improvement are also cheered by realizing that the injury to the child was nutritional and biochemical in origin and is not caused by something the parent had done or neglected to do. Parents of these children so often carry enormous loads of guilt, which psychotherapy has often made heavier.

Dr. Cott believes that hyperactivity in early childhood may be an indication that schizophrenia will occur later in life. In the last part of this extremely important article, he goes into the subject of diet and malnutrition in great depth. And he recounts all the many government surveys which show wide areas of malnutrition among our children as well as adults.

"The universal observations on the dietary habits of brain-injured children, hyperactive children, learning-disabled children and psychotic children have been that these children eat a diet which is high in cereals, in carbohydrate foods and those foods prepared with sugar," Dr. Cott said.

He has carefully studied the blood sugar levels of this group of patients, and he has found an abnormally high incidence of low blood sugar and lack of enough insulin to handle carbohydrates properly. He has also found an abnormally high family history of diabetes in this group.

Turning to minerals, Dr. Cott tells us that little is

173

known at present about our requirements for the trace minerals, and we know even less about all the complex interactions among various trace minerals, vitamins and other food elements. In children who show disorders of blood sugar regulation, he has found disturbances of histamine levels and trace mineral levels as well. In 26 of 30 children he found lower than normal levels of several minerals in analyzing hair for mineral content. Lead was present in every sample tested.

We have been told that the trace mineral zinc is present in ample quantity in our food supply. Today there is evidence this may not be so. Zinc is an important constituent in the body activity that goes on involving chromium, zinc and magnesium, as well as the hormone insulin, essential for regulating blood sugar levels. An excess of other minerals which cannot be avoided may interfere with the body's use of the essential ones. You can readily see how complicated this matter is and how far we can stray from natural, healthful conditions when we begin to tamper with food, taking out some things, concentrating others.

And what of the soil in which the food is grown? Dr. Cott cheerfully takes on the entire chemical and agricultural empire near the end of his article when he says: "Plants grown on a well fertilized soil should contain all the trace elements vital to life. However, the soils of all lands are not adequate, for many of them have been cultivated for a century with fertilizers containing only nitrate, phosphate, potash, calcium and magnesium. These fertilizers grow plants with inadequate levels of trace minerals.

"The use of organic fertilizers or compost provides more of the trace elements," Dr. Cott continued. "The sandy soil of Florida lacks many of the trace elements necessary to grow an abundant citrus crop. At present, zinc, manganese, cobalt, molybdenum, iron and copper salts are all added to the citrus groves." Organic gardening and farming, of course, would solve these problems of trace mineral lack.

Dr. Cott also discusses research in England which seems to show extremely high levels of lead in the blood of city children. He quotes one expert who says that no other toxic pollutant has accumulated in man to average levels so close to the threshold for overt clinical poisoning. Then he tells of another researcher who found that a group of mentally retarded children had distinctly more lead in their blood than a group of normal children. In fact, he says, "nearly half the retarded children had higher blood levels of lead than the maximum level in the other group."

Lead is in the air wherever heavy traffic goes using leaded gasoline. Almost nothing has been done to get the lead out of gasoline, although lots of speeches and promises have been made. We also get lead in food and water. And city children in poor districts who eat flakes of paint from the walls are threatened with lead poisoning if the paint is lead-based.

Summing up his work and the work of others in

treating mentally disturbed children, those who cannot speak, cannot learn, cannot control their hyperactivity, Dr. Cott says: "Investigation of this treatment modality by controlled studies should be given the highest priority, for we are dealing with a patient population of 20 million children."

Subclinical pellagra is what Dr. R. Glen Green calls it in a speech reproduced in the newsletter of the American Schizophrenia Association, July 1970. He describes the symptoms in one 10-year-old girl who was a patient of his. Once bright, interested and alert, she began to complain of abdominal pains and headaches. Formerly an excellent student, she was now getting poor grades. She was cranky, refused to play the piano, once her joy.

Dr. Green examined the girl and could find no physical symptoms which might be causing her troubles. He then began with what he calls "perceptual" symptoms. He asked what words on a blackboard look like. She told him they wriggle around and move back and forth. There is a fog between her eyes and the blackboard. When she looks in the mirror her face becomes bigger, then smaller. Other peoples' faces seem to do the same. The ground moves beneath her feet and buildings appear to be falling on her. She sometimes feels she is not really walking on the ground. She hears voices calling her name. She is afraid of the dark, afraid of school, unhappy and depressed.

Dr. Green began giving her one gram of niacin three times a day. It was given in three doses, because the B vitamins, as is vitamin C, are water-soluble, hence are excreted in the urine, so to keep the body tissues saturated they should be taken frequently.

Within two weeks the child was greatly improved but still had some complaints. By the end of the month, however, she was completely cured and had returned to being her former happy, bright, alert self.

In treating as many as 200 patients suffering from this disorder, Dr. Green says that they notice first that they are tired without reason. They are afraid without reason. They are frightened, depressed and they sleep poorly. Dr. Green asks the patient about perceptual changes. Do things look peculiar or taste bad? Does he have peculiar sensations while walking or lying down? Do things get suddenly big, then little again? He finds, he says, that about 10 per cent of the people who come to him have these troubles, which can be cured almost miraculously by massive doses of niacin.

The sooner the disease is diagnosed, the sooner it can be cured. The less protein there is in the diet, the greater the chance the disease will appear. It tends to run in families. If the patient has had the symptoms for only a few weeks, he can be cured in a few days.

Dr. Green calls this disorder "subclinical pellagra" for several reasons. First, its symptoms are similar to those of pellagra, the disease of nutritional origin resulting from too little niacin in the diet. Although the perceptual symptoms are those of schizophrenia, parents don't want to hear that their children are suffering from a mental disorder. "Subclinical pellagra" sounds better. It doesn't sound too serious and it sounds as if the treatment might be easy. And it is ridiculously easy. One simple vitamin and a high-protein, low-carbohydrate diet is all there is to it.

Dr. Green believes that many inmates in penitentiaries have this disorder and he thinks they are in jail *because* they have it. Children who wet the bed, who do poorly in school, who can't see the blackboard in class, who sleep badly can very often be greatly benefited by taking these large amounts of vitamin B3 and following the prescribed diet.

Said Dr. Green: "Many teenagers have it (subclinical pellagra) but many will not accept treatment. I feel that many of these children are the ones who take pot and LSD trying to find out what is wrong with them."

In a recent report from the Institute for Child Behavior Research, 4758 Edgeware Road, San Diego, Calif. 92116, Dr. Bernard Rimland (Ph.D.) tells of using high doses of vitamins in the treatment of children with severe mental disorders.

"Like most professionals," Dr. Rimland explained, "our training has led us to believe that one's normal everyday diet contains all the vitamins and minerals required, and that anyone advocating the ingestion of larger quantities must therefore be a food faddist, charlatan, stockholder in a vitamin manufacturing concern, or simply naive. Quite probably it is true that most people do not require supplementation of their vitamin intake. The general rules about how much of each vitamin is needed, such as the official Minimum Daily Requirement are no doubt widely applicable. They are clearly, however, not universally applicable. It is individuals who are severely abnormal, who may be possible exceptions to the rules, that concern us. In terms of behavior we are concerned with the three or four most abnormal of each 10,000 children."

Dr. Rimland goes on to say that scientific literature shows that mentally ill individuals do indeed have markedly different ways of using vitamins. By corresponding with various groups and individuals, Dr. Rimland secured detailed records on 57 individual children who had been treated with massive doses of vitamins, some of them on a trial-and-error basis by their parents.

He found, he says, enormous variety in the dosages given. Niacin in one form or another was given in levels ranging from 30 milligrams to 6 grams (6,000 milligrams) a day. Vitamin C, used in 27 cases, was given in doses ranging from 100 milligrams to 6 grams per day; pyridoxine from 5 milligrams to 400. Pantothenic acid was given in amounts from 25 to 900 milligrams.

One California psychiatrist reported on 10 children, saying that some of the results have been "absolutely fantastic." At least half the children treated have shown dramatic improvement. An East Coast physician reported that in treating 50 children, his results have been most encouraging. Still another found results to be very impressive.

Another West Coast doctor, trying vitamin therapy on a 13-year-old schizophrenic, got excellent results up to a certain point, when progress stopped. He inquired at the hospital's pharmacy and found that the boy's prescription for 500 milligram tablets of niacin had been refilled with 50 milligram tablets because of an error. On the higher dosage, improvement began again.

Mothers reported results that sound almost unbelievable—"elimination of tantrums, more alert, more responsive." Still another, "Within a week after starting the vitamins, his behavior at nursery school . . . began to improve. He began to follow orders, became less negative and began to enjoy himself."

One mother reported that when she added massive doses of vitamin C to the prescribed dose of niacin, there was improvement almost overnight that was "fantastic, amazing, unbelievable." A British professor reported that his autistic child had been found to have abnormal metabolism of vitamin B6. Other autistic children (those who daydream or who have hallucinations) who were tested showed the same thing. The professor's child was given pyridoxine and within three months began to improve. His progress seems remarkable.

Most of the children reported on have already been given many psychoactive drugs with little success. Some parents withheld the vitamin therapy to see whether they might be just imagining the improvement. But fears, noise sensitivity, screaming, behavior difficulties and learning difficulties returned almost at once. Going back to vitamin therapy once again brought improvement.

"There is no dearth of research implicating the vitamin metabolism in mentally ill humans," Dr. Rimland said. "We have already referred to the work of Hoffer and Osmond on the use of ascorbic acid and niacin in schizophrenia. A number of other writers have recently published papers showing a highly consistent and quite strong tendency for schizophrenics to fail to excrete vitamin C when it is given in multi-gram quantities (thus indicating that their tissues were not saturated; they needed more). Vander Kamp (1966) found that it required an average of 40 grams (almost 600 times the MDR) per day of oral ascorbic acid before it appeared in the urine of a group of chronic adult schizophrenics, while a control group of normal individuals began to excrete ascorbic acid after only four grams a day (average) has been taken. . . .

"It has been known for many years," Dr. Rimland added, "that one form of severe mental illness in adults, pellagric psychosis (that is, psychosis resulting from pellagra) is caused by a deficiency of niacin, and that the sick person quickly returns to normal upon being given the niacin his body needs. Are there some mentally ill persons, adults or children, whose mental illness may similarly be corrected by adding niacin or some other vitamin to their daily diet? The stock answer has been, 'Giving niacin to a psychotic with pellagra helps him only because his diet lacks niacin. A person with a *normal* diet gets enough niacin to prevent mental disorder, and so will not be helped by additional amounts of the vitamin.' The error in this argument becomes obvious when we consider *atypical* individuals such as a child with vitamin D-resistant rickets. Only massive quantities of the vitamin will help."

Dr. Rimland's paper is available from the Long Island Schizophrenia Association, 1691 Northern Blvd., Manhasset, N. Y. 11030.

CHAPTER 11

An Innovative Medical Textbook on a New Concept of Nutritional Medicine

FOR YEARS many victims of schizophrenia, alcoholism, drug addiction and/or low blood sugar, who have approached their doctors and asked for nutritional help from diet and vitamins, have been told by their doctors or psychiatrists that such a treatment does not exist or that it's just imaginary. Such claims, they maintain, are simply the aberrations of cranks, faddists and opportunists. Now, at last, there is an excellent, complete, authoritative medical textbook available for all physicians and psychiatrists to read.

As we mentioned earlier, it's called *Orthomolecular Psychiatry* and it is a collection of 30 chapters by different specialists in this field. It was edited by Dr. Linus Pauling, one of the giants of modern biology and twice winner of the Nobel Prize, and Dr. David Hawkins, who is mentioned often in this book.

One approaches this 700-page volume with great respect. The authors of these chapters are pioneers in a totally new field of medicine. They have, together, developed and put into practice an entirely new concept of the way the body works. This concept is inherent in the word "Orthomolecular," which was coined by Dr. Pauling. According to this concept, various cells in the body may have widely varying needs for different nutrients. Brain and nerve cells may need much larger amounts of certain B vitamins and vitamin C, for instance, although other parts of the body do not show any apparent nutritional deficiency.

Applying this concept to schizophrenia, alcoholics, drug addicts, etc., the specialists who write the chapters in the Pauling-Hawkins book have, with varying success, been able to achieve almost unbelievable results, regardless of age or length of illness, although, as we have indicated, the sooner the treatment is used, after symptoms appear, the more likely it is to be successful.

The chapter on "Subclinical Pellagra," by Dr. R. Glen Green, who has also already been mentioned in this book, goes to the root of the problem when he says, "As long as people are ignorant, they eat what pleases the taste buds and satisfies the appetite. . . . As long as there are people to whom profit means more than the health of the nation, the poor and the ignorant will be exploited by hucksters peddling puffed wheat, cornflakes and the 'Instant This and That' nearly all at the expense of the protein and vitamin values of the food."

In the section dealing with clinical diagnosis, the physician reader of the Hawkins-Pauling book will discover how to use the Hoffer-Osmond Diagnostic test designed to measure visual, auditory, olfactory, touch, taste and time perceptions, or dysperceptions along with other laboratory tests that can pinpoint schizophrenia in children or adults. Dr. Allan Cott describes his use of a metronome to uncover difficulties in time perception in patients. Their reaction to different settings of the metronome disclose the variations in their time distortions, actual malfunctions which they themselves had begun to believe were imaginary.

In one chapter on testing schizophrenics for certain blood elements, including trace minerals, three scientists from the New Jersey Neuro-Psychiatric Institute bring up the matter of the importance of trace minerals for the health of the brain. Chromium, for instance, is likely to be missing in our diets, due to food processing, yet this is essential for the body to use carbohydrates properly. Part of the schizophrenic's problem is an inability to metabolize carbohydrates. The soil and the trace elements it contains are vitally important to life, especially the brain and nerve cells. But impoverished soils produce food lacking in trace minerals. On the other hand, drinking water piped through copper pipes is likely to pick up enough copper to pose a threat of toxicity. The zinc that we used to get from galvanized pipes may now be lacking in our diets if we have copper pipes.

Patients with zinc deficiency may crave salt, so they oversalt their food, get thirsty, have to drink more water, get more copper in the water, in an unending, unhealthy cycle. Who would ever imagine that a physician's textbook on schizophrenia would discuss such apparently trivial details of living? But, in the orthomolecular concept of mental illness, each of these details assumes immense importance. Who can say whether lack of chromium, for example, may be one of the most important causes of these terrible mental and emotional disorders? How many years will it take us to find out?

In the final chapter on "Orthomolecular Psychiatry: Treatment of Schizophrenia," Dr. David Hawkins outlines, for physician readers, the treatment he has found to be most effective at his Long Island clinic. Every detail is given, so there can be no excuse for failure because of misunderstanding the treatment or the diet or miscalculating the essential dosage of vitamins needed.

Dr. Hawkins tells us that the LSD Service for drug addicts has for years relied primarily on giving megavitamin doses and on attempting to raise blood sugar levels to counteract adverse psychedelic drug reactions. "It is notable that they have discovered that high doses of thiamine hydrochloride (vitamin B1) have been found to be beneficial in reducing the craving and return to the use of methedrine (speed)." This sentence alone may provide us with the knowledge to fight the present drug addiction epidemic, which is destroying so many lives in our cities and suburbs.

Dr. Hawkins goes on to say, "The use of niacin and niacinamide in ameliorating LSD reactions is well known among the more knowledgeable members of the drug subculture and has been reported widely in the underground newspapers. *The Hippy's Handbook* (Bronsteen, 1967) details the use under 'Rx for a Bad Trip' and also has this to say about psychiatry, 'without one single exception, every hippy interviewed had, at one point, gone to a therapist—in every single case the experience was negative . . . modern 'psychiatry is out of touch with young people.' The 'Practical Advice' section of Abbie Hoffman's *Revolution for the Hell of It* (1968) includes similar advice to avoid the psychiatric establishment and to use niacin or niacinamide for 'freak-outs.' The use of megavitamins for the 'drug wipeout' is described in the Do It Now Foundation's *Conscientious Guide to Drug Abuse* (Pawlick, 1971).

"The evidence for the effectiveness of the combination of megavitamins and hypoglycemic diets in correcting perceptual disorders, whether they are associated with outright schizophrenia, alcoholism or drug use, is derived from widespread experience in a variety of patient population groups and settings.

"We can compare the results of this treatment with statistics as given by authorities in the field of schizophrenia," Dr. Hawkins continues. "For instance, the Chief of the Center for Studies of Schizophrenia for the National Institute of Mental Health, Dr. Lorin Mosher, indicates that only 30 per cent of the patients who develop schizophrenia are able to return to work, and according to Coffey et al. (1970), only 15 per cent of patients who had been hospitalized for any appreciable length of time ever function in a completely normal way thereafter. Statistics from New York State Department of Mental Hygiene indicate that 50 per cent of patients hospitalized for schizophrenia are readmissions and in this percentage are many patients with multiple rehospitalizations. As compared to these overall large-scale statistical guidelines, it would appear beyond any doubt that the orthomolecular psychiatric approach offers substantial and valid hope to patients and family. As the number of patients increases, the development of an integrated community system for the treatment of schizophrenia evolves to meet the growing needs of the patient population. The strength of the system, however, relies entirely on demonstrable results."

The Hawkins-Pauling book was certainly not written for the average lay reader. It is a medical textbook for physicians and psychiatrists. But if you have problems of this nature in your family or in your neighborhood, suggest to the people involved that there *is* another way than the usual psychiatric treatment—a way based on nutritional common sense and a new concept of the way the body uses nutritional substances—the orthomolecular concept. Ortho means optimum or best. Thus, "orthomolecular psychiatry" means treatment of mental illness based on the best possible physical environment for the mind. Now, for the first time, the record of achievement with this treatment is available for the medical profession—in this monumental book which, we firmly believe, may change the course of history by changing our outlook on the cause and treatment of these many widespread disorders.

Orthomolecular Psychiatry, edited by David Hawkins and Linus Pauling, is published by W. H. Freeman and Co., 660 Market St., San Francisco, Calif. 94104. The price is $17.00. It contains 92 illustrations and 79 tables.

CHAPTER 12

Are You a Victim of Low Blood Sugar?

"ADDICTIVE PEOPLE SEEM to have one thing in common: an underlying hypoglycemia. We certainly see hypoglycemia in sugar addicts, in alcoholics, in coffee addicts. People who have studied hard-drug addicts report to me that hypoglycemia is common among them. Cola beverages have long been addictive for many people," states Dr. Robert C. Atkins in his new book, *Dr. Atkins' Diet Revolution,* which we will have more to say about later.

Low blood sugar (also medically known as hypoglycemia or hyperinsulinism) is roughly the opposite of diabetes. And specialists in this field believe that low blood sugar is directly related, not only to alcoholism and drug addiction, but also to epilepsy, asthma, multiple sclerosis, rheumatic fever, peptic ulcer, nervousness, fatigue, some forms of mental illness, allergies, etc.

In diabetes, it is thought that the body does not produce enough insulin—a secretion of the pancreas, which helps the body to use sugar and other carbo-hydrates—so that levels of sugar become so high that sugar may overflow into the urine. The pancreas is a large, somewhat elongated gland that is situated behind the stomach. It also secretes a digestive juice (pancreatic juice) into the small intestine.

Low blood sugar is exactly the opposite. The body glands manufacture too much insulin, so that blood sugar levels are entirely too low most of the time. Since many important functions of the body—chiefly those involving the nerves and the brain—depend upon sugar in the blood, they may actually become sugar-starved in such a condition. Obviously, such a state may have serious consequences.

The diabetic may be given a manufactured in-sulin to make up for the secretion which he can-not produce himself. If he gives himself too large a dose, he may suffer from insulin shock: perspiration, great nervousness and anxiety, trembling, fatigue and possibly even death. Babies whose mothers are diabetic may die of insulin shock in the womb.

If the low blood sugar patient goes too long on an inadequate diet or too long without eating at all, he may induce much the same kind of condition in himself—or the symptoms may take on a number of bizarre forms. He may get irritable, even violent. He may develop terrible headaches. Or, as we have mentioned, he may become neurotic, alcoholic or a drug addict. In any case, these disorders may be the aftermath of several years of low blood sugar levels.

If these diseases are caused by too little sugar in the blood, the best diet to overcome them might seem to be a diet rich in sugar. In the early days of experimentation, doctors used to give their patients sugar when they found that hypoglycemia was present. They gave them candy or glucose tablets to eat whenever they felt the symptoms of low blood sugar returning.

For a time this seemed to work, until, gradually, the patients found that they needed the sugar supplements almost all the time. They kept them on bedside tables and ate them whenever they awoke during the night; they carried them about during the day and ate them constantly. If they did not, the unpleasant and dangerous symptoms returned shortly after meals.

Those are the two key words to hypoglycemia: "after meals." Symptoms are always improved by eating—no matter what. But when the meal is loaded with sugar and starch, symptoms return after several hours or perhaps less. So the doctors took another look and decided to try a different kind of diet.

Perhaps the same diet prescribed for diabetics would work for hypoglycemics, too. Sure enough, a diet high in protein, with sugars and starches omitted or cut to a minimum, and with a moderate amount of fat, steadied the wild swings in blood sugar readings so that the badly affected patient could eventually go from breakfast to lunch without any symptoms, from lunch to dinner without any complications. He was essentially cured. And the diet was approximately the same diet a diabetic would have to follow.

The spacing of meals is important to a hypoglycemic, as it is to the diabetic. He must eat frequently. In the diet prescribed by Dr. Seale Harris —and later made famous in the excellent book, *Body, Mind and Sugar,* the low blood sugar patient must take four ounces of fruit juice or an orange or grapefruit immediately upon arising, eat a high-protein breakfast, take four ounces of juice two hours after breakfast, a high-protein lunch, then eight ounces of milk three hours after lunch, and four ounces of juice an hour before dinner. After a high-protein dinner, he must take eight ounces of milk within 2-3 hours, then four ounces of milk or a small handful of nuts every two hours until bedtime.

By "high-protein" diet we, of course, mean the following: meat, eggs, fish, milk, cheese, and other high-protein foods in normal quantities, plus all vegetables except potatoes, and all fruits except those mentioned below. They may be cooked or raw, with or without cream—but without sugar.

Only one slice of bread or toast may be eaten at any meal; spaghetti, rice, macaroni and noodles are forbidden. Salad greens of all kinds, mushrooms and nuts may be eaten as often as desired.

For beverages, any *unsweetened* fruit or vegetable juice (except grape or prune juice), weak tea, decaffeinated coffee, coffee substitutes, club soda, distilled liquors are allowed.

Absolutely forbidden on the diet are: sugar, candy

and other sweets such as cake, pie, pastries, sweet custards, puddings and ice cream; caffeine—either as strong tea, coffee or soft drinks containing caffeine; potatoes, rice, grapes, raisins, plums, figs, dates, bananas, pasta foods, wines, cordials, cocktails and beer.

An added word is perhaps necessary about the caffeine. Dr. E. M. Abrahamson, the physician co-author of *Body, Mind and Sugar,* tells us in his book of patients whose blood-sugar regulating mechanism was so sensitive to caffeine that even one cup of coffee would undo the benefits of weeks of painstaking dieting.

If you are such a person, you would do well to substitute decaffeinated coffee or some other beverage for coffee, because, apparently, there is no hope of your being able to drink coffee or strong tea without inviting a low blood sugar crisis. And that almost inevitable companion of a cup of coffee—the cigarette—will also lower your blood sugar.

It is easy to see that the daily routine followed by millions of Americans is creating nutritional cripples insofar as blood sugar levels are concerned. The individual who eats no breakfast, as we often remind you, or takes only coffee or coffee and something sweet, then lights up a cigarette, has started the vicious cycle.

Within an hour or so, his energy is ebbing, his nerves are on edge, he's tired, restless. It's coffee-break time. The combination of caffeine, a sweet bun and another cigarette shoots his blood sugar levels up to a new high. He feels fine for a short time. But soon the levels are plunging down again and the symptoms return. If he skips lunch or eats a lunch consisting mostly of carbohydrate, he will have another period of fatigue, jitters, nervousness, restlessness or possibly headache in the late afternoon. If he takes another coffee break, with some easily assimilated carbohydrate, the symptoms may recur again before dinnertime.

At dinner he gets the sugar-regulating mechanism back to normal for a time with some protein food, but, if he has been eating this way for years, the blood sugar levels may swing wildly down again by bedtime. They will reach their lowest point during the night or early morning.

By breakfast our patient is grouchy, headachy, tired. He may even be trembling and faint. The breakfast coffee and cigarette bring the blood sugar up and restore him—but not for long. As the situation becomes worse, the periods of comfort grow shorter and shorter. After the first time he has blacked out at the wheel of his car, the sufferer will have to see a doctor.

So many physicians refuse to recognize the existence of a diet-induced condition such as low blood sugar that a foundation— Adrenal Metabolic Research Society—has been organized to publicize this condition and combat it. The group is headed by individuals who got into health trouble themselves because of a diet that led to low blood sugar. Working alone and without the financial backing most national health organizations have, they are doing a good job of spreading the word about hypoglycemia. Perhaps there is a chapter in your area.

Incidentally, you have noticed that the list of forbidden foods on the low blood sugar diet includes such excellent foods as figs, dates, raisins, plums, bananas, etc. This does not mean that these are harmful foods—only that they should not be eaten while one is trying to re-educate all the complicated mechanism of glands and digestion involved in the low blood sugar condition. After you have the mechanism regulated, you can, of course, begin to take these foods again—in moderation.

Homeostasis is the word most often used by Dr. John Tintera in describing what he tried to obtain in his treatment of alcoholics with diet and gland therapy. Homeostasis is defined as the maintenance of a "steady state" by coordination of all physiological systems. In Dr. Tintera's work, the steady state was achieved by treating the blood sugar regulation mechanism and also by giving certain hormones which rejuvenated the adrenal glands.

As long ago as 1956, Dr. Tintera wrote in the *New York State Journal of Medicine* (December 15) that alcoholism is a symptom of a glandular disorder. Taking alcohol will temporarily relieve the deficiency, said Dr. Tintera, but it increases the stress under which the alcoholic is laboring and aggravates the condition so that uncontrollable drinking results. Giving adrenal cortical extract, Dr. Tintera produced dramatic results, he said, in rehabilitating the alcoholic. At the same time, he prescribed the diet which corrects low blood sugar.

In an article in *The Journal of the American Geriatrics Society* (February 1966), Dr. Tintera stated that malnutrition and lack of vitamins have been pinpointed as the basic cause of alcoholism for many years. But why should prosperous individuals, with plenty to eat, suffer from such a condition? "One reason," he says, "is that many of these people continue the onslaught against the adrenals by substituting readily available carbohydrates for the alcohol. Even so, others who follow the low-carbohydrate, moderate-fat, high-protein diet may be relieved of such symptoms as the 'dry jitters' (hypoglycemia crisis) but still suffer from other mental and emotional symptoms due to an erratic blood sugar level. . . . It is common to find A.A. members carrying a candy bar or a lump of sugar to be ingested in case they have an attack of the dry jitters. If left to their own resources, recovered alcoholics naturally adopt a diet high in carbohydrates. In no instance have we found these patients to be free of hypoglycemia. The hypoglycemia is preceded by hyperglycemia (high blood sugar) the severity of which depends upon the amount and duration of damage imposed upon the liver and adrenals through the consumption of alcohol and, later, carbohydrates. Indeed, Banting once stated that more cases of hepatic cirrhosis are produced in hard soft-drinkers than in hard hard-drinkers."

By far the most important part of the treatment of alcoholics is the complete restriction of easily absorbed carbohydrates, said Dr. Tintera. Vitamin

C is essential because the adrenal glands need it for efficient functioning, and it is the adrenal glands which are so terribly deranged in the alcoholic. But preventing low blood sugar episodes is as important as vitamin C. A low fasting blood sugar is found after meals in *all* untreated, recovered alcoholics, he reports. The adrenal glands, incidentally, are two small ductless glands on the upper part of the kidneys. They are also known as the suprarenal glands.

Dr. Tintera's theories on blood sugar disturbances and adrenal exhaustion are available for both the layman and the physician in material you can get from the Adrenal Metabolic Research Society of the Hypoglycemia Foundation, Inc., P.O. Box 98, Fleetwood, Mount Vernon, New York 10552.

They include such titles as: *What You Should Know About Your Glands, What You Should Know About Your Glands and Alcoholism, Hypoglycemia and Me?* and much material on the high-protein, low-carbohydrate diet. There is also an interesting pamphlet entitled, *Delinquent Glands Not Delinquent Juveniles.*

"Don't wait for children to become dropouts," this latter pamphlet pleads. ". . . They can but don't do well in school—they have bursts of energy and excessive periods of 'laziness' and 'disinterest.' They eat poorly, especially at breakfast and frequently crave sweets and use lots of cola or other soft drinks. . . "

Young drug addicts can also be restored to good health through the program which this Society describes in its literature. Write to them for lists of the materials they have available. Some of the treatment must be administered by your doctor. The diet and vitamin supplements are safe for anyone to use, whether or not their doctor sees any sense to it.

The high-protein, low-carbohydrate diet that Dr. Tintera suggests is, as to be expected, similar to the diet that we discussed earlier in this chapter. Peanuts and soybeans, on his list, are high in carbohydrate, but he apparently feels that their protein content will insure the patient that the carbohydrate is released so gradually during the digestion process that little damage can be done to the blood sugar regulating mechanism. And the kinds of foods that Dr. Tintera recommends have their own built-in guarantee against over eating.

Here is Dr. Tintera's diet list:

Foods Allowed

All meats, fowl, fish and shellfish.

Dairy products (eggs, milk, butter and cheese).

All vegetables and fruits not mentioned below.

Salted nuts (excellent between meals).

Peanut butter, oat and jerusalem artichoke bread.

Gelatin with whipped cream.

Sanka, weak tea and sugar-free soft drinks.

Soybeans and soybean products.

Oatmeal.

Certain high-protein macaroni and spaghetti.

Foods to Avoid

Potatoes, corn, macaroni, spaghetti, rice and cereals.

Pie, cake, pastries, sugar, candies.

Dates, raisins and other dried fruits.

Cola and other sweet soft drinks.

Coffee and strong tea.

Alcohol in all forms.

Dr. Bernard Rimland, whom we have mentioned in an earlier chapter, who treats schizophrenic children in his San Diego, California clinic, had this to say about sugar:

"Sugar and sugar-containing food provide, as you know, empty calories. Children who should be eating meat, fish, cheese, nuts and other protein foods are instead gorging themselves on candy, cupcakes, cookies, punch and the like. They are thus not only taking in dangerous sugar but simultaneously failing to eat real food. And one strong sign of relative hypoglycemia is an almost insatiable craving for sweets."

Dr. Rimland also believes that allergies are related to mental illness. He says, "Until recently few seem to have realized that the most sensitive organ in the body, the brain, is also vulnerable to malfunctioning if someone eats and drinks the wrong substances. There is a strong and important division of opinion in the medical profession on this topic. Nevertheless, the evidence for food-caused allergies of the nervous system is impressive and convincing."

Again and again the word "hypoglycemia" appears in medical literature about alcoholism. *Annals of Internal Medicine* for July 1963 tells of a woman who drank only "sporadically." Three times she went into hypoglycemic coma—that is, coma brought on by blood sugar too low to support brain activity.

"A history of very low food intake with recent high alcoholic consumption was obtained" each time. No one knows what causes these conditions, according to the two physicians who wrote the article. Perhaps the alcohol damages the liver's ability to process sugars and starches. Perhaps there is an inherent abnormality of carbohydrate metabolism. In every case, an injection of glucose brings the patient back to normal, just as it would bring a diabetic back to normal.

The Journal of the American Medical Association, October 14, 1968 reported on five cases of diabetics brought to the hospital in deep coma because they had been drinking. Three of the five had permanent damage to the nervous system and the other two died without recovering consciousness. The Harvard physicians who treated them point out the necessity of explaining to diabetics that alcohol lowers blood sugar and this must be taken into account by diabetics who are taking insulin or diabetes drugs to control swings of blood sugar levels.

A Parisian doctor reports in a French medical journal on a study of blood sugar regulation in 60 patients with chronic alcoholic liver diseases. Blood sugar disorders were extremely common, he says. Ninety per cent of those studied were abnormal, of which 58 per cent were the diabetic type. There was a correlation of the severity of the liver disease with the blood sugar disorder—the worse the blood sugar picture, the worse the liver disease.

A 1970 study of blood sugar levels in rehabilitated alcoholics showed that there are definitely metabolic abnormalities in these people, meaning that biochemical and inherited factors are probably causing their alcoholic problems. The doctors found abnormally high levels of lactic acid in the blood of some of the patients, low blood sugar in others. Dr. Lawrence Rutter believes that overactivity of the adrenal glands produces anxiety in some people. Injecting small amounts of lactic acid produces much more anxiety. Non-alcoholics can deal with this amount of lactic acid without any trouble. But alcoholics cannot.

Three Swedish doctors, writing in the *Lancet* for January 20, 1968 say they have observed two types of disturbances of carbohydrate metabolism in chronic alcoholics with liver disorder. One kind has a diabetic type of inability to deal with sugar. The other has low blood sugar. So both diabetes and low blood sugar occur in alcoholics.

Back in 1964, a specialist in the study of alcoholism was telling the public that "the alcoholic has a peculiar sensitivity to alcohol. According to the newest theory, the alcoholic reacts to alcohol in somehow the same way that the diabetic reacts to sugar." According to *The New York Times*, June 21, 1964, Dr. William Keaton said that in each group of 13 people who drink alcohol, 12 can take liquor and get a certain form of relaxation from it. "The 13th person's drinking may not differ from the others in its early stages, but after a while something will happen that sets off a chain reaction in him. Although he may not consume more alcohol than some of the other 12, it will become a disease for him."

Not many physicians think of sugar addiction as being a true addiction. Here is the testimony of one British doctor who does. It's from the *Lancet* for April 6, 1963.

"Patterns of overeating vary from person to person. My problem was sugar added to cereals and beverages. To my own concern and that of my wife, I discovered I was consuming two pounds of sugar a week in this form, and that the amount was rapidly increasing. Part of this was the result of a lifelong 'sweet tooth.' I had always been fond of sweet things because of their taste. But a disturbing feature about my recent craving was that it was increasingly powerful and progressive. If fought, it resulted in most unpleasant symptoms.

"On stopping beverage and cereal sugar," he continued, "I suffered from sweating, abdominal pains and a liability to syncope (fainting). My mental condition was impaired, and I had headache and subjective head noises. My temper was uncertain. I was continuously apprehensive and very difficult to live with. These symptoms were immediately relieved by taking sugar. If withdrawal continued, the symptoms settled within two weeks; but it would be disagreeable to repeat the experience.

"In summary, I was eating more and more sugar, and its withdrawal caused the intensely unpleasant symptoms of endogenous hyperinsulinism (another name for low blood sugar). I was caught in a vicious circle. My problem was not excess weight, but true sugar addiction. The discovery of this fact caused me to revise my psychological attitude. Sugar was now to be regarded as the enemy—always there, always to be guarded against. A brief period of dieting was not enough; I was an addict, and I had to live with my addiction permanently.

"Thinking of this kind is not over-dramatic," the English doctor said. "It is an entirely practical down-to-earth approach, which in my case has removed 2 stone (about 28 pounds) of unnecessary weight, and which has proved very useful for my patients with the same complaint. Obesity is produced by many factors, but sugar addiction like mine cannot be rare. In such cases, if my own experience is any guide, telling the patient not to overeat simply produces a tolerant smile.

"But tell the patient he is an addict to sugar, and his reaction will be very different. The very phrase conjures up to him the seriousness of his position, and the necessity for a lengthy and continuous campaign—not to take off his excess poundage but to reorganize his whole mental attitude towards his very real problem."

Thus, there seems to be ample evidence that addiction to sugar and all other excessively sweet foods may be at the heart of all addiction in susceptible people.

Dr. Norman Freinkel believes that drinkers who appear to be "dead drunk" or in an alcoholic coma are actually in a coma caused by low blood sugar. Examining nine such patients in a hospital emergency room, he injected glucose and recovery was rapid. Later he injected alcohol equivalent to three or four shots of whiskey and found the same result—

almost immediate recovery. Dr. Freinkel believes that it is the alcohol itself which produces this reaction in susceptible people. The longer such people go without food the more severe the low blood sugar reaction will be.

One pathetic, and extremely important note from a *New York Times* article (August 1, 1972), discussing the drug addiction of Alan King's son: "The lean figure in the flared corduroy hip-huggers sat at the table in the dining alcove of his upper East Side apartment and shoveled sugar into his coffee." Later in the interview he drinks another cup of coffee, presumably with the same enormous load of sugar.

In April 1973, another of King's sons was turned in to the police by his father for allegedly possessing marijuana and hashish. In an interview in the *New York Post*, April 16, 1973, King said that the other son, "is completely rehabilitated and works in a drug rehabilitation program trying to help other youths."

"(My son) was supposed to be on marijuana," King said. "But as liberal as I may think I am, nobody can tell me that marijuana is the same thing as booze was during prohibition. I know through my involvement in the drug scene . . . what marijuana leads to."

Two significant comments on fructose were made in a 1965 issue of *Medical World News*. A University of Copenhagen physician showed that taking fructose when you are drinking helps the body to get rid of alcohol harmlessly. Fructose is a fruit sugar. This may explain why drinks mixed with tomato or fruit juice tend to cause less distress on the "morning after" and why juices might alleviate the distress at that time.

In the same issue of the magazine, we are told that fructose cuts the insulin requirement of diabetics. A New York physician gives 25 to 50 grams of this fruit sugar to "brittle" diabetics (the kind that require careful and continual control) along with oral diabetic drugs. Within three weeks, some of the diabetics required no more insulin, while others needed much smaller amounts. The wild "swings" from high to low blood sugar were avoided and blood sugar levels were steadied.

Dr. Benjamin P. Sandler of the Departments of Medicine and Pathology, Veterans Administration Hospital, Oteen, North Carolina, has published a number of books and papers on hypoglycemia. For example, in 1940, he published a paper in *The Review of Gastroenterology* on how to control the pain of ulcers with a low-carbohydrate diet. A paper on chronic abdominal pain due to low blood sugar, and another on the low-carbohydrate diet in controlling angina pectoris, the pain of a certain heart condition, were published in 1941.

More recently, Dr. Sandler treated a patient with subacute bacterial endocarditis with a high-protein, low-carbohydrate diet, while he was administering antibiotics, and he reports that the patient's temperature was normal within 24 hours and his blood showed "early and persistent" decrease in bacteria. Dr. Sandler says that the diet played an important role in the patient's rapid recovery from the fever.

How to Prevent Heart Attacks is the title of a book

that Dr. Sandler published in 1958. Although it was not a book on reducing, there is ample evidence relating heart attacks and obesity, and Dr. Sandler says that patients who eat his suggested diet lose weight if they are overweight and gain weight if they are thin.

Since 1937, as Dr. Sandler points out in his book, he has performed hundreds of tests on patients to look for low blood sugar tendencies. And he reports that he has found evidence of low blood sugar levels in more than half of them. He also has found that a diet planned to correct the low blood sugar either eliminated or alleviated many symptoms not only in patients whose blood sugar levels were low, but also in those who appeared to have normal levels. "I have concluded that any human can experience low blood sugar as long as he or she consumes sugar and starch," Dr. Sandler says.

Continues Dr. Sandler: "I regard as artificial the rapid rise in blood sugar level produced by eating foods containing sugar. The sugar is an artificial stimulant; and, in some people, the desire for sweets amounts to a craving and the demand for something sweet during this craving amounts to an addiction.

"I regard this craving for sweets as abnormal," he continues. "The low blood sugar that comes on around 11 a.m. is due to eating sugar or starch at breakfast, and the low blood sugar at 4 p.m. is due to eating sugar and starch at the noon meal. On a high-protein, low-carbohydrate diet the fall in blood sugar at 11 a.m. and 4 p.m. does not occur and so there is no physical letdown and no need for a pick-up. Cigarette smoking can also serve as a pick-up because nicotine can cause an immediate rise in blood sugar level by stimulating the adrenal-sympathetic system, the rise occurring at the expense of liver glycogen.

"The desire for a cigarette actually coincides with a fall in blood sugar and the feeling of satisfaction that comes with a smoke is due to a rise in blood sugar," Dr. Sandler explains. "Denicotinized cigarettes do not satisfy because they do not cause a rise in blood sugar."

Dr. Sandler also says that coffee, tea or cocoa not only cause a rise in blood sugar—by reason of added sugar—but also because they contain caffeine or related chemical compounds that stimulate the adrenal-sympathetic system and thus cause a rise in blood sugar at the expense of liver glycogen.

It is Dr. Sandler's contention that the low-carbohydrate diet is as helpful to the person with low blood sugar as it is to the person who is a diabetic. In either case, the diet regulates the levels so that wide fluctuations are done away with. Consequently, the heart is assured of adequate delivery of sugar at all times and is not exposed to sudden, unexpected lowering of the blood sugar, he says. This sudden lessening of the supply of sugar to the heart is the leading cause of heart attacks, Dr. Sandler feels. And he produces some very convincing cases to justify his claim. In most cases, symptoms of pending heart attacks are relieved by following the recommended diet. The symptoms return when the diet is broken and a few teaspoons of sugar or a few slices of bread are added at every meal.

Dr. Sandler's comments on smoking not only give a graphic picture of what happens when you smoke —both after meals and on an empty stomach—but also he recommends the best possible way of giving up smoking. His simple theory: regulate your blood sugar levels with a low-carbohydrate diet and you will find that you do not crave a cigarette.

The effects of psychological stresses on blood sugar levels are also dealt with. Unpleasant news may send the levels down; sudden emergencies or shocks or heavy work (such as shoveling snow) may deplete the blood of necessary sugar. While the urge to eat something sweet or to drink coffee is strong, the only sensible thing is to eat some protein, which stabilizes the blood sugar levels and protects us to some extent against stress.

"I have found that a diet completely free of sugar and starch and consisting of proteins, fats and non-starchy vegetables, may be adhered to for years with beneficial effects and absolutely without harmful effects," Dr. Sandler says. "There is no supporting evidence to indicate that sugar and starch are necessary for health or for energy purposes. The human is a carnivore and can thrive on protein and fat alone."

Dr. Sandler's diet, as is to be expected, is similar to the others mentioned in this book. All animal foods can be eaten in *unlimited quantity* . . . any meats, fish or poultry—fresh, canned, smoked or dried. Eggs can also be eaten in unlimited quantity, as can all dairy products. Fresh fruits are allowed, but only one portion should be eaten at one meal, since they contain quite a bit of sugar. Fruit juices, canned fruits, dried fruits and preserved fruits are taboo. Fruits can be stewed without sugar; apples can be baked without sugar. Tomato juice can be taken freely, since it contains no natural sugar.

These carbohydrate foods can be eaten in unlimited quantity: artichokes, asparagus, avocados, bamboo shoots, string beans, wax beans, soybeans, red beans, broccoli, brussels sprouts, cabbage, cauliflower, celery, chard, collards, cucumbers, eggplant, endive, greens of all kinds, kale, kohlrabi, leeks, lettuce, mushrooms, okra, onions, parsley, parsnips, fresh peas, peppers, pumpkins, radishes, rhubarb, rutabaga, sorrel, spinach, summer squash, tomatoes, turnips, watercress, pickles, horseradish, mustard, vinegar, olives, capers and mayonnaise.

The following foods, high in carbohydrate, should be eaten in reduced quantity: dried beans (baked, for instance), lima beans, tapioca, macaroni, rolls, crackers, corn, dried split peas, potatoes (white or sweet), yams, lentils, rice, spaghetti, vermicelli, noodles, all breads, buns, biscuits and cereals.

And these foods should be avoided entirely: sugar, soft drinks, ice cream, ices, sherbets, cakes, candies, cookies, wafers, pastries, pies, fruit juices, canned and preserved fruits, jams, jellies, marmalades, puddings, custards and syrups.

"Diabetic foods and desserts" are permitted. Coffee, tea, cocoa, lemonade, etc., may be sweetened

with artificial sweeteners. Nuts are allowed in unlimited quantity, except for peanuts, cashews and
chestnuts, which should be eaten sparingly.

A typical menu suggested by Dr. Sandler is as
follows:

Breakfast: Fresh fruit or tomato juice, two or more
eggs, if desired, plus ham, bacon, fish, cheese or
other meat; no more than one slice of bread with
butter. A beverage without sugar.

Lunch: Tomato juice or soup with no starchy
fillers, as much as you want of meat, fish or poultry
and any of the permitted vegetables, with no more
than one slice of bread and butter; one piece of
fresh fruit and beverage.

Dinner: Similar to lunch with added salad and
nuts and cheese, together with a piece of fresh fruit.

"The high calorie way to stay thin forever" is
the subtitle of the new book, *Dr. Atkins' Diet Revolution*, which we have already mentioned. As was
to be expected, the book, the No. 1 non-fiction best-
seller in the United States as this is being written,
has had the medical profession and practically all
orthodox nutrition experts rolling up their sleeves
and preparing to engage in verbal battle with an
author who would dare to suggest that anyone can
lose weight by any method but counting calories.

Dr. Atkins, who has a private practice in New
York, tells us that he has treated about 8,000 overweight patients with a diet which might total 5,000
calories a day. And they all lose weight satisfactorily.
He has had no failures; he has had no unhappy

reports of faintness, weakness, fatigue, irritability. Instead, his patients tell him they have never felt better. They are wide awake, full of energy, never hungry.

Dr. Atkins has carried the "Calories Don't Count" diet several steps further. For the first week or so, his patients are allowed to eat nothing but protein and fat—that is, their meals are confined to foods which contain no carbohydrate. They eat meat and eggs, plus salad greens with lots of salad dressing. They lose weight immediately; they feel better immediately.

Here are some sample menus. For breakfast, scrambled eggs with ham; for lunch, cold cuts with mayonnaise or mustard; for dinner, chicken soup and steak; for a snack, a vegetarian bacon product. And there is no limit—you can eat all you want of these.

In addition, you may have measured amounts of foods which contain a smidgeon of carbohydrate: rolls or bread which contain no flour (recipes are given for these); salads with plenty of oil and vinegar, diet sodas and gelatin desserts made with synthetic sweeteners. This is a typical menu for starting on the diet. One of his patients lost 100 pounds eating 4½ pounds of meat a day.

As you progress and lose weight, you are permitted to add carbohydrate-rich food—little by little—if you wish, stressing those things you miss most in the way of starchy foods. When you reach a certain point, which Dr. Atkins calls your individual "Critical Carbohydrate Level," that's where you stay. From then on, you plan meals to include, for you, no more carbohydrate than that—ever!

You are overweight, says Dr. Atkins, because your body is unable to deal successfully with carbohydrate foods. So, for the rest of your life, you must eat no more than this level of carbohydrate, in grams. The kind of carbohydrate food you choose is up to you, but it must contain no more than the number of carbohydrate grams which correspond to your Critical Carbohydrate Level.

Discussing his patients' inability to use carbohydrate foods gets Dr. Atkins into discussions about diabetes and low blood sugar which, he says, are two aspects of the same disease. The people who start out with low blood sugar will probably become diabetics. Diabetes, low blood sugar and overweight go together naturally, since all of them are caused by the body's inability to use carbohydrates.

You might ask, how does it happen that so many of us—perhaps half of all Americans—have problems with one or more of these conditions of ill health? As has been a leitmotif throughout this book, Dr. Atkins believes all the trouble can be blamed on the refining and processing of high carbohydrate foods. Even more important was the single event which probably led to more illness than any other thing in history—the discovery of how to refine sugarcane into white sugar. Dr. Atkins hates sugar with a passion. And he justifies this feeling on every page of his most convincing book.

But you will never be hungry again. If you want

to go on an eating binge, this is perfectly permissible, any time of the day or night. But you must eat only foods that contain protein and fat—eggs, meat, fish, poultry, cheese.

You can eat in any restaurant and Dr. Atkins tells you how. You just skip the dishes on the menu that contain carbohydrate and have as much as you wish of the others. If a food is unfamiliar, ask the waiter if it contains starch or sugar. If it does, order something else. Leafy green salads are permissible any time, anywhere.

The recipes and menus in the last part of the book were devised by former patients of Dr. Atkins. The meat, cheese, fish, egg and poultry recipes are fine—the kind of thing all of us should be eating every day. The diet "bread," crackers and rolls are made with eggs, cottage cheese, soya powder and a bit of synthetic sweeteners and products made from them.

Dr. Atkins' patients are mostly people with intractable problems of overweight. They have tried everything; nothing works. But they invariably lose weight on his diet. And Dr. Atkins says that, without fail, their cholesterol counts go down, as well as the levels of other fatty substances in their bloodstream. He says that it is because, on this diet, with all or most of the carbohydrate fuel removed, the body must consume its own fat cells. And that is what brings about weight reduction without any discomfort or hunger.

If you omit all fruits and many vegetables from your everyday meals, where will you get your vitamin C? Dr. Atkins believes that you need large amounts of this vitamin. He, therefore, requires his patients to take up to one gram (1,000 milligrams) of vitamin C daily. He also prescribes 800 milligrams of vitamin E routinely to every patient. He finds, he says, that vitamin E appears to have a beneficial stabilizing effect on blood sugar levels. If they are too high, it brings them down. If they are too low, it brings them up.

We urge you to read this book, whether or not you have a problem with overweight. The material on diabetes, low blood sugar and addiction is invaluable. And it is all explained in easy-to-understand terms.

Sid Caesar, the actor and comedian, reported on his reducing diet in a recent issue of the *Ladies Home Journal.* He has had such a problem with overweight that he told the *Journal* that the diet with which he took off 50 pounds and reduced his waistline eight inches is the diet he must follow the rest of his life. This is agreeable to him. He has no complaints about the diet; he feels better, thinks better, looks better, works harder than ever before. *And he never counts calories.*

"Going on my diet is like quitting cigarettes," he said. "I know it's forever. My diet will work for most normal, healthy people, because it provides the essential vitamins and nourishment. . . . What I've given up in quantity, I've made up in quality. I eat only the best meats, fruits and vegetables. . . ."

There's a new cookbook called *The Low Blood Sugar Cookbook,* by Francyne Davis (Grosset and

Dunlap, New York, $6.95), who is a low blood sugar victim and who developed these recipes for her own family table. On the one hand, we feel that any cookbook designed for the low blood sugar patient is unnecessary. As we have stated, make your meals mostly one main course of meat, fish or poultry, plus a low-carbohydrate vegetable and a big salad; prepare everything as simply as possible.

The egg, poultry, fish and meat dishes in Mrs. Davis' book are just about what you would find in any cookbook. You bake or roast, broil, fry or saute without adding pasta or potatoes or beans or any of the other high-carbohydrate foods. Vegetables and salads are also just about what you would find in any cookbook, except that the high-carbohydrate vegetables are omitted. Tasty recipes for spinach, string beans and summer squash (all on the recommended list, of course) are welcome, certainly, and this cookbook has them.

Unfortunately, the last half of the book consists of desserts made with artificial sweeteners, and, although some of the experts we have quoted in this book recommend artificial sweeteners, we think that recommending desserts made with them is a serious mistake. We believe that, as long as the hypoglycemic continues to persuade himself that he must have a large quantity of something with sweet taste at the end of a meal, he is much less likely to get over his problem with sugar than those of us who deliberately choose a dessert of cheese and nuts or a piece of raw fruit. So we deplore the idea of a low-carbohydrate diet embellished with loads of desserts, even though they are made with artificial sweeteners. Why not, instead, get totally away from the idea of dessert and eat so much good, hearty, high-protein food at every meal that you simply have no room for desserts of any kind?

Mrs. Davis recommends oat flour rather than wheat flour, apparently with the mistaken impression that oat flour contains more protein and less carbohydrate. It does not. And wheat germ, which she could have used instead of oat flour in many recipes, contains immense amounts of protein and relatively little starch.

Nor do we see any reason for advising the hypoglycemic that, "should your doctor permit you chocolate in small quantities, buy only unsweetened baking chocolate." True, it contains only 7.7 grams of carbohydrate per ounce, but what chocolate addict ever stopped at one ounce? Stay away from chocolate! Stay away from any foods that remind you of the gooey, sticky, sugary goodies you used to eat. Those are the foods—every one of them— which got you into this condition in the first place.

We also see no reason why Mrs. Davis should warn against corn oil. No salad oil contains anything but fat. There is no carbohydrate in any of them, so why discriminate against corn oil? With these few reservations, we recommend Mrs. Davis' cookbook. Most valuable, perhaps, are the Introduction by Marilyn Hamilton Light, Executive Director of the Adrenal Metabolic Research Society and the Foreword by Carlton Fredericks, as well as a good first chapter on the general dietary program, some suggested menus and "Helpful Hints" at the back of the book, with information on what to buy and what not to buy.

Many health store products are recommended: soy flour, toasted soybeans, cooked and canned soybeans, raw soybeans, pasta made from artichoke flour (the carbohydrate in this is not absorbed), oat flour, water-packed fruits, bouillon, fruit concentrate syrup with no added sugar, etc.

Judge Tom R. Blaine, a state district judge in nine Oklahoma counties, has written a book, *Goodbye Allergies*, in which he described the way he cured his own lifelong allergies with a diet and injections of adrenal extracts. In the process of following the diet (which is the same high-protein diet used to treat hypoglycemia), Judge Blaine became absorbed in the subject of low blood sugar and its possible relation to other disorders in addition to allergies.

In his professional life he had dealt with many disturbed human beings, many criminals, alcoholics, schizophrenics, drug addicts. Is it possible, he asked himself, that the reason for some of these terrible personal tragedies may be simply an unsuspected low blood sugar condition? He began to do research on the subject, corresponded with many professional leaders in fields of psychiatry and medicine, who were already using the diet in the treatment of many assorted emotional, physical and mental illnesses.

Finally, he wrote another book, *Mental Health Through Nutrition*, dealing with "Hypoglycemia, the Ignored Disease," "Vitamins Bring Mental Health,"

"Schizophrenia Responds Favorably to Vitamin Therapy" and many related subjects. The evidence he· has collected is a formidable indictment of modern diets, loaded as they are with refined foods and white sugar. Judge Blaine's facts come from many corners of the earth. All are well documented. He gives names and titles of the people he quotes. Because he is a judge, rather than a professional scientist or physician, his writing is easy for the layman to follow. There are no complex biological terms or concepts. There is extensive information about the diet for treating low blood sugar and how to follow it.

Judge Blaine has turned up some information not generally available in most books on the subject. He says, for example, "Dr. Joseph Wilder of New York, specialist in psychiatry and neurology, found that low blood sugar is far more serious with children than it is with adults. Dr. Wilder said, 'The importance of nutrition for mental functioning is much greater in children than in adults. In adults, faulty or insufficient nutrition may alter or impair specific or general mental functions, and eventually cause reparable or even irreparable structural damage of the central nervous system. In children, we face a grave additional factor. The development of the brain may be retarded, stopped, altered, and thus the mental functions may become impaired in indirect and not less serious ways. . . . The child may be neurotic, psychopathic, and be subject to anxiety, running away tendencies, aggressiveness, a blind urge to activity and destructiveness, with impairment of moral sensibilities. . . . In its simplest form, it is a tendency to deny everything, contradict everything, refuse everything, at any price.'" Does this sound like anything you read in your newspapers or see on TV . . . such as widespread drug abuse, the alarming number of suicides among teenagers, etc.?

The book, of course, does not deal only with youth. Judge Blaine is aware that, as we grow older, there is a tendency toward eating less nutritious diets and to reward ourselves with more empty calorie sweets. The aging brain and nervous system need protein, vitamins and minerals in perhaps even larger amounts than younger persons need. And he tells us stories of near miracles worked in old folks with good, nourishing diet and plenty of vitamins and minerals.

The sections on schizophrenia are enlightening. Judge Blaine includes letters from patients and their families describing their condition before and after treatment with megadoses of vitamins and the diet to correct low blood sugar. These are patients of Dr. Abram Hoffer, Dr. Humphrey Osmond and other pioneers in the use of this kind of treatment for schizophrenia. His book is well provided with names and addresses of helpful organizations in this field, names and addresses of physicians who use this treatment, books to read, professional books to get your doctor to read, and several valuable appendices with information on vitamins, minerals and so on.

It's a fine beginner's book on the subject of the

dietary treatment of low blood sugar and the use of megadoses of vitamins for treating many emotional and mental disorders. *Mental Health Through Nutrition,* by Judge Tom R. Blaine, is published by Citadel Press and priced at $5.95. *Goodbye Allergies* is published by the same firm; in paperback for $2.00; in hardcover for $5.95.

According to some authorities, you inherit your tendency to be allergic. If your mother and father both are allergic, there is a 50 per cent chance you will be, too. There is a 57 per cent chance of allergy in children who have only one allergic parent. About 15 per cent of modern Americans are allergic to some one thing or many things. Another 25 to 30 per cent are less easily sensitized. About 55 to 60 per cent never have allergies.

Says Richard A. Kern, M.D., in *Archives of Environmental Health,* "The allergic person is born that way and so remains until he dies . . . He may have eczema in infancy, hay fever in adolescence, then asthma in middle years, and finally eczema again in old age—all of these caused by different allergies." Dr. Kern goes on to describe allergy as a disease of modern times which has steadily become more prevalent as more potential allergenic substances are introduced in our environment. Every new chemical, drug, household product or commercial process is bound to cause someone, somewhere to react allergically. Hunting down and eliminating these allergies becomes more difficult with every passing year.

According to Dr. Kern, primitive people seem to have fewer and less severe allergies than "civilized" man. He presents a fascinating theory which may help to explain this. He describes the Norway rat which has been used in laboratories for more than 100 years. Considering the life span of the rat, this corresponds to 5,000 years in human history. Some time ago a researcher named Richter decided to examine some Norway rats whose ancestors had been living in laboratories and compare them to wild Norway rats. He found that the adrenal and pituitary glands were much smaller in the laboratory rat—the adrenal cortex being only about one-third of the size of the corresponding organ in the wild rat.

It is difficult to make a rat allergic to anything. To do so one must remove most of the adrenal gland. So it appears that this gland must have some important bearing on one's susceptibility to allergies. The wild Norway rat needs a full-size adrenal gland so that he can get away from his enemies or fight them to the death if he is cornered. The Norway rats whose ancestors have lived in a quiet laboratory where there are no enemies and no stressful situations have, over many generations, lost most of their adrenal glands. They don't need them, for they never encounter situations where they have to fight or run.

Says Dr. Kern, "One is tempted to believe that man, like the captive Norway rat, has had to fight less and less for his existence and so has less and less need for his 'fight' and 'stress' mechanism, with a consequent reduction in size and function of his

adrenals." Primitive man—much more free of allergies—still lives as he has for centuries, surrounded
by all the enemies that have always threatened him.
He still needs the power his adrenal glands give him
in an emergency to fight or flee. Could the size of his
adrenal glands be one reason for his comparative
freedom from allergies?

A recent United Airlines study seemed to demonstrate that Federal Aviation Agency medical examinations are not sufficient to guarantee that all
U.S. pilots are in physical condition to pilot planes.
Dr. Charles R. Harper gave the exams because of
reports of working pilots struck with attacks of low
blood sugar.

Some of the incidents involved tingling in the
arms and legs, weakness of arms and/or legs, blind
spots combined with flashing lights in their eyes, and
mental confusion during certain kinds of aerial
maneuvers. Another pilot showed "poor airmanship
and judgment" during an approach to a landing field
and had to crash-land. "In both pilots," says *Medical
World News* for October 27, 1972, "an oral glucose
tolerance test indicated precipitous drops in blood
glucose (sugar) along with behavioral and physio-
logic aberrations."

Dr. Harper began his study in 1969 to discover,
if he could, which other pilots might have symptoms
of low blood sugar. Out of 175 pilots over 40 years
of age, 44 showed a disconcerting drop in blood
sugar at the first examination. But they reported no
other symptoms. At the end of the second year, 30 of

these 44 reported episodes of drowsiness, poor thinking, irritability, tremor, faintness and various digestive troubles. One pilot admitted that he sometimes had to pull his car off the road because he felt "mentally confused."

All of the pilots were put on a low-carbohydrate, high-protein diet "with plenty of unsweetened fruit", according to the *News*. The diet worked. None of the pilots was grounded. The Vice President in charge of medical services said he had no idea why these pilots should have such a tendency. He was certain it could not be caused by "stress."

There are, of course, many different definitions of "stress." One would think that long hours without sleep or rest, without food or with inadequate food, which may, we suppose, be the lot of at least some pilots would be the very "stresses" most likely to bring on symptoms of low blood sugar.

We were puzzled to read in a recent issue of *Newsweek* a statement by a medical man that many physicians view the current "flurry" over hypoglycemia as somewhat overblown since, after all, "it may be just the result of poor eating habits," hence it may require only an adjustment in the diet.

Why adjusting the diet is viewed as something inconsequential is a mystery to us, since it appears that correct diet and eating habits are the single most important aspect of living which contributes to good health. Apparently, many doctors may feel that low blood sugar isn't very important as a health threat, since there is no drug they can give to "cure" it instantly. But, as we have demonstrated time and time again throughout this book, low blood sugar is at the root of many of our most damaging disorders.

CHAPTER 13

Is Low Blood Sugar Related to Aggression and Violence?

A STARTLING NEW theory proposed by a young anthropologist associates low blood sugar with violence and aggressive behavior. Dr. Ralph Bolton of Pomona College, California, recently returned from Peru, where he spent five years living with the Qolla peasants in a remote mountainous area.

Dr. Bolton believes he has found a connection between the hostile, aggressive behavior of these Peruvians and low blood sugar levels. This is a condition which can masquerade as many different physical diseases, as we have discovered throughout this book.

The Qolla have no problems with reducing diets. Instead, like poor people in the United States, they suffer gross dietary deficiencies from eating a low-protein, high-carbohydrate diet, consisting mostly of potatoes, barley, oats and guinua, a grain which will grow at high altitudes. In addition, they live in a very hostile environment. The terrain is hilly, mountainous and barren. The climate is erratic, with hail, drought and frost, which means that harvests are likely to be uncertain and scanty.

Dr. Bolton describes the Qolla as people who enjoy a good fight, because "it makes one feel better." Very hostile and aggressive, these two million people are pretty regularly "spoiling for a fight" just for the heck of it. The anthropologist believes that the combination of circumstances—inadequate diet, overpopulation, scarcity of land, unpredictable weather and lack of enough oxygen (because of the altitude at which they live) may be the starting points for the development of low blood sugar levels.

He found the Qolla to be "strutting, swaggering individuals" especially when they are drunk. They will go to outrageous lengths to insult others and precipitate a fight, sometimes indulging in monologues "describing their own ferocity while laughing at the puniness of their enemies." Threats produce such sensitivity in the Qolla that just the phrase "you'll see" can be construed as a verbal attack. Saying "I am a man" immediately implies that others are not men, so whoever is within hearing distance takes this sentence as an insult and a battle ensues.

Fighting and killing are not the only forms of aggression. Injuries, insults, stealing, rape, arson, abortion, slander, failure to pay debts, land ownership disputes and homicide are common. In one village of 1,200 Qolla, Dr. Bolton found that half of the heads of households had been involved, directly or indirectly, in homicide cases. The rate of homicide among the Qolla is 50 per 100,000—far higher than in almost any other group in the world.

Surprisingly enough, the traditional philosophy of the Qolla is far from aggressive. They believe in the Christian virtues of charity, compassion and cooperation with others. And they almost never perceive any discrepancy between their beliefs and their actions. Other anthropologists have always found the Qolla to be "the meanest and most unlikeable people on earth." Traditionally, this has been excused on the basis of the extreme hardness of their lives and the fact that they have usually lived under domination by one or another conquering nation.

Dr. Bolton believes this is not the complete story. Other nations living under harsh conditions do not have the same characteristics of aggression and hostility. True, the Qolla have been conquered many times, but, he says, they tend to ignore outside influences, even conquerors, and continue to go about their own hostile pursuits. They live in a constant state of anarchy.

The anthropologist had read about hypoglycemia and decided to test some of the Qolla. He did blood sugar analyses of all adult males in one village and found that blood sugar levels were low in 50 per cent of them. Another interesting factor is that they chew the coca leaf. *Encyclopedia Britannica* tells us that coca leaves are the substance from which cocaine is made. Their action is similar to that of opium, though somewhat less narcotic. They deaden the sense of taste and anesthetize the membranes of the stomach, thus cutting off hunger.

So it is possible, under the influence of coca, to go without food or consciousness of needing it for as long as three days. But the body starves, as might be expected. Continual heavy use of coca produces body wasting, mental failure, insomnia, circulatory weakness and dyspepsia. However, under the influence of the drug, addicts are able to perform great feats of endurance.

In addition to chewing coca leaves, the Qolla use a lot of alcohol, again, Dr. Bolton believes, in an effort to bring blood sugar levels up to a comfortable condition. Alcohol does this in susceptible persons, then causes these levels to drop far below normal, bringing on the same symptoms the alcoholic has tried to overcome. So it becomes necessary to have another and yet another drug of some kind, merely to keep going with any comfort.

Very little research has been done on low blood sugar in relation to aggression. During the 1940's, a number of American doctors proposed the theory that low blood sugar is the leading cause of many acts of criminal violence—even murder.

Hypoglycemia may be a factor, says Dr. Bolton, in some cases of criminal behavior in so-called "civilized" societies. An otherwise normal-appearing person may be driven to commit atrocities by his body's urge to restore a proper blood sugar balance. Aware that the body will go to extraordinary lengths to repair a malfunction within itself, Dr. Bolton believes that the Qolla are forced into aggressive behavior by their physical condition.

Dr. Bolton is convinced that, through aggressive

thought and activity, the Qolla unconsciously try to raise their blood sugar levels to a comfortable point. Psychologically they force themselves into a state of anger so their internal organs can temporarily restore a proper bodily balance.

He further believes that hypoglycemia should be suspected when studying social conflict and behavior patterns of any "peasant" culture. We wonder why he specifies "peasant" since many of the circumstances he outlines appear to be just as prevalent on city streets, where badly nourished people commit crimes just to get money for drugs, where apparently sane people go berserk within hours of apparent sanity and kill wildly and indiscriminately anyone they can reach with a gun.

Dr. Bolton goes on to say, "The question of peasant personality generally should be looked at again, since many of the same factors which serve as stressors for the Qolla are present in most peasant societies. Research on this topic might be carried out in American ghettos and other poverty areas where high levels of stress are found."

Dr. Bolton does not mention it, but, obviously, one form of stress on city streets must be the low blood sugar caused by a deficient diet overbalanced with sweets and carbohydrates, especially the concentrated sugar involved in soft drinks and candy, which, as we have mentioned often in this book, make up such a large part of the diet of so many people.

Dr. Bolton plans to go on studying this line of thought. His study opens up, he says, many research possibilities—for example—detailed studies of the relationship between coca chewing and other drug use and hypoglycemia, the relationship between alcohol consumption and hypoglycemia, and the consequences of hypoglycemia for other psychological processes, such as perception, memory and cognition. He believes, too, that a study of aggressive societies and peaceful ones may lead eventually to a significant anthropological contribution to a general theory of human conflict and aggression.

A full account of Dr. Bolton's work will be published soon by National Press of Palo Alto, California. It is called "Aggression in Qolla Society."

We would like to point out that, in primitive Eskimo societies, conditions of environmental stress are also extreme. The cold, the darkness, the continual battle for food must indeed be among the most difficult ways of life anywhere in the world. However, primitive Eskimos eat a diet consisting almost entirely of protein and fat. Carbohydrates are unknown except for a few short summer days when berries and other vegetable foods are available. Diet the year around consists of meat and fish, with large amounts of fat.

Primitive Eskimos are so far removed from aggressive behavior that there is no word for "war" in any Eskimo language. In fact, explorers have described trying to make their Eskimo friends understand what is meant by war. The Eskimos simply refuse to believe that any human being could possibly go out and kill total strangers for any reason. We know of no studies of blood sugar levels among primitive Eskimos. But it appears that they must be very well regulated, since this kind of diet practically guarantees this.

As we have mentioned, we occasionally hear reports of various investigations by resourceful scientists of the possible relationship between crime and poor nutrition. Obviously it is difficult to sort out all the many environmental elements that enter into the personality of any one person. Someone who commits a serious crime is no exception. Probably both heredity and home, school and community environment are responsible to some degree for the type of individual who is driven to commit murder, armed robbery, rape, etc.

An Egyptian physician, writing in *Schizophrenia*, the newsletter, believes that the lack of an essential B vitamin may have a great deal to do with the personality of the criminal. Dr. El Kholy studied crime and pellagra from 1941 to 1948. Pellagra, as we already know, is the disease of a niacin or vitamin B3 deficiency. Protein is also lacking in the inadequate diet that produces the disease.

Dr. Kholy, as do many researchers in this field, maintains that pellagra can easily be mistaken for a schizophrenic personality. He examined 1,150 people who had been accused of serious crimes. He found that 206 or 18 per cent had pellagra. Their crimes included murder, threats to kill, attempted murder, serious assault, kidnap, arson, rape, etc. Over one-third of all who were later declared to be insane murderers were found to have pellagra.

The newsletter goes on to make these comments: "Had pellagra been prevented, there would have been a major decrease in crimes of violence.

"Here the psychiatrist finds an important parallel between pellagra and schizophrenia. Both conditions, he states, are clinically so similar that they have been, and are, easily confused. Both respond to treatment with vitamin B3, although psychiatrists who have not used the megavitamin B3 approach still deny this, and both can be prevented by adequate intake of vitamin B3. . . . As a rule patients who have recovered from schizophrenia and are well physically and mentally will not relapse while taking adequate doses of either nicotinic acid or nicotinamide.

"By analogy, if elimination of pellagra reduces crimes of violence, how much more will eradication of schizophrenia achieve? It is suggested, therefore, that perhaps the addition of nicotinamide to our food in doses of one gram per day or more will do for schizophrenia what the fortification of flour with much smaller doses of nicotinamide has done for pellagra."

While on the subject of crime, we are reminded that Dr. R. Glen Green is confident that many inmates in the penitentiary have subclinical pellagra, and he thinks that they are incarcerated *because* they have this disorder.

How long must we wait until further research along these lines brings to light the seriousness of the problem of low blood sugar in our population and its relation to crime and violence of many kinds, as well as its relation to alcoholism, drug addiction and another condition where a different kind of addiction is involved—obesity and overweight?

CHAPTER 14

Coffee Drinkers, Beware!

Two NEW BITS of research on the modern American addictions came to light recently in experiments with rats given coffee and other experiments where the animals were given alcohol in amounts comparable to those consumed by many of us prisoners of an urban technological society.

Two University of California scientists gave coffee to rats, then studied their blood pressure. They found that coffee may produce its harmful effects on blood pressure and heart when it is drunk in lively company with a crowd of others, but not when it is taken alone.

Isolated rats, living alone, were given coffee in large amounts. They showed no rise in blood pressure, almost no heart damage. Rats from the same families living peacefully together were given the same amounts of coffee. At once they started to fight and developed sharp increases in blood pressure and heart damage.

A third group of rats, already aggressive and fighting among themselves, became even more so when they were given a similar amount of coffee. Their blood pressure shot up, heart damage increased. The blood pressures were taken of animals given water, decaffeinated coffee and real coffee. The blood pressure was 134 on water, 143 on coffee. In a group living crowded together, blood pressure was 126 on water, 130 on decaffeinated coffee and 164 on full-strength coffee.

Dr. James P. Henry, who conducted the studies, said that coffee of itself does not affect blood pressure. But when it is accompanied with the stimulus of community life, the stimulation is the key factor. Coffee increases the intensity of reactions, including excitability. "It is, of course, well known that amphetamines are more lethal when given to groups than when given to isolated animals," he said, "and if you are a cool individual who does not get excited, you can drink all the coffee you want. But in a society with so many uptight people as this, I don't think we can all normally afford to do this."

People who drink more than five cups of coffee a day have about twice the risk of having an acute myocardial infarction as those people who drink no coffee at all. So, at least, we are told by two physicians at Boston University Medical Center, who collected data on the daily beverage intake before hospital admission of 276 patients with this kind of heart attack.

Then they compared this group to 1,104 controls who were patients with other diseases. They asked all the patients if they usually drank none, or one to five or more than five cups of coffee daily and also how much tea they drank.

Comparing the two groups, they found no significant differences in tea consumption in the two groups. In fact, while the heart attack patients consumed more coffee than their controls in the nonheart attack group, they consumed a lot less tea.

There seems to be a consistent relation between drinking lots of coffee and having heart attacks in both young and old people. This was true for those who also had diabetes and high blood pressure, two conditions often linked with heart attacks.

The two physicians, Dr. Hershel Jick and Dr. Dennis Stone, think personality may have something to do with the situation. Possibly, they theorize, patients who drink lots of coffee and have heart attacks have similar personalities, so that is the main reason—not the coffee drinking. They have no proof either way on this. It's also possible, they think, that there is some substance or substances in coffee other than caffeine that makes people who drink lots of coffee more susceptible to heart attacks. They rule out both caffeine and added sugar as having anything to do with the problem, since tea drinkers get as much of both of these as coffee drinkers do. And have fewer heart attacks. It is also interesting that the heart attack victims were big smokers.

What other possible reasons might there be? Well, maybe people who had previous heart attacks could have increased their intake of coffee as a reaction to the stress of having a heart attack. There is no data available to prove or disprove this theory. This research, incidentally, was reported in the January 6, 1973 issue of *Science News*. It was initially reported in the December 16, 1972 issue of *Lancet*.

The Surveillance Program which was responsible for conducting this study is now working on another, more ambitious one involving some 600 patients.

In his book, *Vitaminology*, Dr. Walter Eddy mentions a curious fact about the possible relation of inositol deficiency and drinking too much coffee. Inositol is a B vitamin. When laboratory animals were given large amounts of caffeine, a paralysis occurred which could be cured by giving them inositol. So possibly caffeine may have some destructive effect on this vitamin-like substance.

Whether or not you happen to be the "personality type" which just might be more liable to heart attack than the rest of us, doesn't it seem a good idea to cut your intake of coffee as low as possible?

Your health food store offers the largest collection of beverages you may wish to use in place of coffee. First, there's plain water. If you live in a city and your water is so loaded with chemicals you can't bear to go near the stuff, you can always buy bottled spring water. Then there are coffee substitutes of many kinds: decaffeinated coffee, which is at the moment under a bit of suspicion as being not so much better than regular coffee, though nothing has been proven as yet.

Then there are herb teas, well over 100 of them. There are the coffee substitutes generally made from cereals. You brew them very much like you would brew coffee and drink them with cream or milk, plus a bit of honey, if that's the way you like them. And how about a carob drink for breakfast? Use carob powder added to hot milk. Drink milk, buttermilk or soybean milk.

Get a blender and mix yourself highly personalized blender drinks involving fruit or vegetable juices, plus milk or buttermilk or yogurt, plus some powdered seeds or nuts for added protein. Or get acquainted with fresh raw vegetable juices made in a juicer. Almost any vegetable, from parsley to carrots to lettuce, can be made into a fine, tasty juice with the flick of a switch in any of the convenient, modern juicers.

Or, of course, you can buy canned or bottled juices of almost any variety in your health food store. Fruit juices range from the very familiar to the exotic and unknown. Try them. Try some of the many vegetable juices. You'll find they are filling, rich in vitamins and minerals, more satisfying than plain water and, of course, completely healthful. Skoal! Here's to your health.

CHAPTER 15

Smoking Disorders Blood Sugar Levels

WOULDN'T IT HAVE been wonderful if the ultimate in sophistication, sexuality and sinfulness, instead of being cigarettes, liquor—and now pot—had been, say, a fresh apple, a bowl of grapes or maybe a slab of unprocessed cheese on a slice of black bread? But as soon as Hollywood's super-stars began to flaunt their drinking and smoking with increasing regularity on the silver screen, teen-agers by the millions, from Maspeth to Manilla, rushed out of the theater to emulate their movie idols. And once they became hooked, they continued these vices into adulthood, resulting in nothing but zeroes in the health column.

And some of the proponents of Women's Lib, who should know better, seem to think that the epitome of equality is to be able to smoke cigars and cigarettes and to drink in bars. Consequently, Dr. Donald Kent, medical director of the National Tuberculosis-Respiratory Disease Association, reports that cigarette usage for women has climbed during the past 15 years, while that for men has dropped. The number of women dying from emphysema and chronic bronchitis has doubled in the last decade, he added.

U. S. Public Health Service statistics show that, in 1955, 59.9 per cent of U. S. adult males smoked cigarettes. In 1970, the percentage had dropped to 42 per cent. During the same period, women smokers increased from 28.4 per cent to 31 per cent.

There was a 6.5 million increase in the number of men who quit smoking from 1966 to 1970, compared to only 3.8 million women, stated the National Tuberculosis-Respiratory Disease Association, 1740 Broadway, New York, N. Y.

The Association does not have statistics as yet for 1971 and 1972, but the U. S. Department of Agriculture predicted in September 1972 that per capita smoking would average 204 packs for Americans over 18 in 1972, compared to 202 in 1971, or the most cigarette use in four years, according to the *New York Post*, November 30, 1972.

Dr. Daniel Horn, director of public services of the National Clearing House on Smoking and Health, said that, "until recently, women have had to resist cultural pressure more than men if they were to smoke. Women fought harder to smoke and have held on to the habit more tenaciously."

Helen Jones, an associate director of the National Tuberculosis-Respiratory Disease Association, stated that women, more than men, were afraid of gaining weight if they stopped smoking. A free pamphlet is available from the Association which offers tips to women on how to stop smoking and not gain weight.

There is strong evidence that pregnant women who smoke cigarettes are increasing the risk of death of their babies, according to *The New York Times* for January 18, 1973. The announcement was made by the Public Health Service.

"Twelve retrospective and prospective studies have revealed a statistically significant relationship between cigarette smoking and an elevated mortality risk among the infants of smokers," the PHS report stated.

The document also raised doubts concerning the safety of the small cigars that are now in vogue. "Many people can inhale these in the same way they do cigarettes, and those who do will probably face increased risks of the lung and heart problems that have been linked to cigarette smoking," the PHS continued. The PHS also stated that smokers of pipes and large cigars face some health risks, too.

"The Health Consequences of Smoking, a Report of the Surgeon General, 1972," a 158-page document, is available for 70 cents from the Superintendent of Documents, U. S. Government Printing Office, Washington, D. C. 20402. Ask for Report #1723-0051.

Speaking at a news conference at the American Cancer Society's 59th annual meeting, at the Waldorf-Astoria Hotel in New York, October 24, 1972, Dr. Luther L. Terry, the former Surgeon General who released the first reports linking cigarette smoking and cancer, said that he would like to see all cigarette advertising banned. He said that, since the government's prohibition of cigarette advertising on radio and TV began in 1971, the tobacco industry has diverted most of its promotional material to newspapers, magazines and billboards.

He added that he is also concerned about the increase in broadcast advertising of "little cigars," which are mild enough to be inhaled like cigarettes. There is no ban on cigar advertising. Dr. Terry's remarks were reported in the October 25 issue of *The New York Times*.

Meanwhile, the commercial stake in cigarettes and alcohol is apparent if you check on the advertisements that appear in magazines in general circulation. For example, *Time* magazine, for December 18, 1972 (the pre-holiday issue) carried 70 pages of advertising, of which 33 were for either liquor or cigarettes.

"Cigarette smokers who droop their cigarettes from their lips instead of holding them in their fingers run a far higher risk of developing chronic bronchitis, according to a report in the *British Medical Journal*," said the *New York Post*, March 30, 1973. The report was based on a survey of over 5,000 cigarette smokers who attended a mass chest X-ray in Southeast Lancashire in 1970-71.

According to the *Post*, 8 per cent of those surveyed smoked their cigarettes without removing them from their lips. Of the normal smokers, 33 per cent had symptoms showing they were developing chronic bronchitis; and, of the droopers, 41 per cent had these symptoms. Although not mentioned in this study, the droopers are also probably more susceptible to lip cancer.

Continued the *Post*: "The droopers tend to breathe more 'sidestream' smoke—that which comes directly from the burning end and is not filtered through the cigarette—the report says. And it says this smoke probably contains more tar than 'mainstream smoke' —the kind that goes through the tobacco."

Another item in the *Post*, this one in the March 29, 1973 edition, states that a medical researcher, Dr. Wolfgang Vogel, says marijuana apparently is likely to produce cancer as cigarette tobacco does because pot-smokers usually hold the smoke in their lungs as long as possible.

Dr. Vogel and his associates have studied marijuana with the same testing procedures used in the study by the U. S. Surgeon General that linked cigarette smoking to cancer. Dr. Vogel and his colleagues at the Veterans Administration Hospital in Coatesville, Pa., have spent several months studying 60 mice in the tests. Twenty of the mice that received an application of a solution containing marijuana tars on their skin for five days developed signs of cancer, according to a spokesman for Thomas Jefferson University.

"True, nobody smokes 20 reefers a day, but the smoke from each puff is deliberately held in the lungs for as long as possible, unlike the case with cigarettes," the *Post* quoted Dr. Vogel as saying. "You can probably get as much tar from two reefers as you would from a pack of cigarettes."

Most of us are more conscious these days of the importance of maintaining normal blood sugar levels. Some researchers believe that the most important aspect of blood sugar regulation is not whether it is too high or too low all the time, but the rapidity with which it swings from one to the other.

Our bodies tend to be healthiest when they do not have extremes to deal with—too much heat or too much cold, too much fatigue, too much food, too little exercise, etc. Given time, however, they can usually adjust to these disadvantages. But when the changes are sudden and frequent—hot one minute and cold the next, no food one week and too much food the next—our bodies have great difficulty making the adjustments.

Blood sugar levels which are too low in the morning, then shoot up to a point much too high after coffee and cigarettes, then drop way below normal before lunch present too great a challenge to our glandular network which must somehow compensate for these wide swings in blood sugar levels and make adjustments throughout all other mechanisms which are interrelated with blood sugar.

Did you know that the smoke from one cigarette —even if it is not inhaled—exerts a tremendous influence on blood sugar level? A Swedish physician, writing in the October 30, 1965 issue of the *Lancet*, reports on experiments which were conducted in 1929 in Sweden. About 100 tests were done on 10 healthy volunteers who smoked cigarettes at varying intervals, so that their blood sugar could be measured before and at varying periods after each smoke.

In the case of one young woman who smoked four cigarettes in a morning, her blood sugar level rose from a healthy 97 or 99 to 111 or 114 and finally to 118 for the last cigarette smoked. The rise in this last case occurred in seven minutes. It represented an increase of 36 per cent.

The Swedish investigators also did tests on de-nicotinized cigarettes and found that they did not affect the blood sugar levels. However, cigars produced the same effect as cigarettes. So the nicotine seems to be responsible.

Says the Swedish doctor who reported these tests, "Very few seem to be aware of this truly spectacular effect of smoking. . . . The effect of the 'hunger cigarette' is easily explained by the rapid rise of blood-sugar, which also explains the increased craving for tobacco in times of war and famine. The rapid fall of the blood-sugar level after smoking throws further light on the habit of chain smoking—the craving for another pick-me up. . . ."

In other words, excessive and long-continued cigarette smoking may possibly result in such disorder of the blood sugar regulating mechanism as to produce diabetes or chronic low blood sugar, which, as we have learned, is the opposite of diabetes. This is a very delicately adjusted mechanism which responds to the eating of sugar as well. We also know that caffeine in large amounts upsets blood sugar levels.

Many people who have tried to give up smoking complain that they immediately put on weight. They are trying, you see, to deal with a blood sugar mechanism already disordered by nicotine, so they eat whenever they would formerly have lit a cigarette. If these snacks are high-protein foods, chances are that the nicotine addict, if he is not too far gone in addiction, can gradually bring his blood sugar levels back to normal and the craving for cigarettes will disappear completely and painlessly. But all too often the smoker is also a coffee, candy and soft drink addict as well. So even though he stops smoking, with a terrific effort of will power, he continues to eat candy, drink soft drinks and coffee and his blood sugar levels continue their wild swings from high to low, while his waistline steadily expands.

The answer for the person who wants to stop smoking is to omit everything that disorders blood sugar levels: cigarettes or cigars, coffee and any food containing large amounts of sugar. He should also nibble frequently throughout the day—but only on high-protein foods like cheese, milk, nuts, seeds, hard-boiled eggs, bits of cold meat, etc. It sounds incredible, but on this kind of diet the craving for nicotine, for caffeine and for sugar can be overcome completely and painlessly within 10 days to two weeks.

The Swedish doctor continues in *Lancet*: "In the very lively discussions of late years on factors causing coronary (heart) disease, excessive carbohydrate (sugar) consumption has been increasingly incriminated as by Yudkin (Professor at a London university), who also incriminates smoking. It seems that in these discussions the blood-sugar raising effect of tobacco has been largely overlooked."

And a London doctor, writing in the November 6, 1965 issue of *Lancet*, said: "More people are attempting to give up cigarette smoking, and some are receiving advice to replace this habit by eating 'mints' and other similar sweets under the misapprehension that these are less injurious to teeth than chewing toffees. I should like to report here a case which will illustrate the point.

"Eighteen months ago a 20-year-old man who was dentally fit gave up cigarette smoking and began the habit of mint-sucking. He recently presented (himself) with over 50 carious lesions (decayed holes) in his teeth. X-rays taken 18 months ago and at the recent examination confirm this transformation. Many may not be aware of the devastation this particular kind of sweets can create in an otherwise healthy mouth."

It's too bad the young man's physician hadn't suggested snacks of sunflower seeds, unsalted peanuts, protein wafers, apples, cheese, celery, carrots, walnuts, etc. He would have overcome his craving for nicotine and would have developed even stronger teeth, since all these foods promote tooth health.

As long ago as 1952, American researchers knew that nicotine added to a sample of whole blood in a test tube decreased the vitamin C content of the blood by 24 to 31 per cent. In 1941, a German scientist demonstrated that vitamin C levels are much lower in the blood of heavy smokers than in the blood of those who do not smoke. And Dr. W. J. McCormick, a Canadian researcher, says that the cigarette smoke inhaled from one cigarette neutralizes about 25 milligrams of vitamin C. So the second cigarette of the day would just about rob us of our daily quota of vitamin C, assuming we had that much to begin with.

In the March 9, 1963 issue of *Lancet*, three scientists described their experiment with smokers and vitamin C. They said they have confirmed that vitamin C is destroyed in a test tube when tobacco smoke comes in contact with it. They tested an equivalent amount of air and the smoke from burning cigarette papers and found that neither of these destroys vitamin C. So it must be the nicotine.

There is also evidence that one eye disorder caused by smoking or drinking is nutritional in origin. *Amblyopia* is a condition where vision is dim, with no organic reason for it. According to a writer in *Archives of Ophthalmology* for September 1963, there is no convincing evidence that this condition is the direct result of poisoning by nicotine or alcohol. Rather, said the researchers, "it is concluded that the primary cause is probably nutritional."

A South African physician, writing in *Lancet*, October 19, 1963, stated that tobacco amblyopia is cured by vitamin B12, even though the individual goes on smoking and even though his blood levels do not indicate that he has any deficiency in this vitamin.

The Journal of the American Medical Association, April 28, 1969, told of experiments in Canada which link smoking to a lack of vitamin C. The research was done by Dr. Omer Pelletier, who conducted his experiments with the assistance of the Canadian Food and Drug Directorate.

Thus, we have seen throughout this book that improper dietary rules, along with excessive use of alcohol, drugs, coffee, tobacco, etc., lead to a vicious cycle of mismanagement, resulting in many kinds of degenerative disorders. As Dr. Albert Szent-Györgyi said earlier: "What I find difficult to understand . . . is not why people become ill, but how they manage to stay alive at all."

Suggested Further Reading

Abrahamson, E. M. and A. W. Pezet, *Body, Mind and Sugar*, Pyramid Books, New York, 1971.

Adams, Ruth and Frank Murray, *Body, Mind and the B Vitamins*, Larchmont Books, New York, 1972.

Adams, Ruth and Frank Murray, *Is Low Blood Sugar Making you a Nutritional Cripple?*, Larchmont Books, New York, 1971.

Adams, Ruth and Frank Murray, *Vitamin C, the Powerhouse Vitamin, Conquers More Than Just Colds*, Larchmont Books, New York, 1972.

Atkins, Robert C., M.D., *Dr. Atkins' Diet Revolution*, David McKay Company, Inc., New York, 1972.

B.H.C. *Description, Diagnosis, Theory and Treatment of Schizophrenia*, Karpat Publishing Company, Cleveland, Ohio, 1972.

B.H.C. *Hope Giving Stories of Schizophrenic Patients*, Karpat Publishing Company, Cleveland, Ohio, 1972.

B.H.C. *Low Blood Sugar*, Karpat Publishing Company, Cleveland, Ohio, 1971.

Blaine, Judge Tom R., *Goodbye Allergies*, The Citadel Press, New York, 1965.

Blaine, Judge Tom R., *Mental Health Through Nutrition*, The Citadel Press, New York, 1969.

Brecher, Edward M. and Editors of *Consumer Reports, Licit and Illicit Drugs*, Little, Brown and Company, Boston, 1972.

Cheraskin, E. and W. M. Ringsdorf, Jr., *New Hope for Incurable Diseases*, ARCO Publishing Company, New York, 1971.

Davis, Francyne, *The Low Blood Sugar Cookbook*, Grosset & Dunlap, New York, 1973.

Fredericks, Carlton, *Low Blood Sugar and You*, Constellation International, New York City, 1969.

Hawkins, David and Linus Pauling, *Orthomolecular Psychiatry, Treatment of Schizophrenia*, W. H. Freeman and Company, San Francisco, Cal., 94104, 1973.

Hoffer, Abram, M.D., Ph. D., *New Hope for Alcoholics*, University Books, New Hyde Park, New York, 1968.

Hoffer, Abram, M.D., Ph. D. and Humphrey Osmond, M.R.C.S., D.P.M. *How to Live With Schizophrenia*, University Books, New Hyde Park, N.Y., 1966.

Megavitamin Therapy and the Drug Wipeout Syndrome, an Introduction to the Orthomolecular Approach as a Treatment for After-Effects of Drug Use/Abuse, Compiled by Vic Pawlak, Director, Do It Now Foundation and Do It Now Staff, P.O. Box 5115, Phoenix, Arizona 85010. Price, 35¢ each.

Megavitamin Therapy in Orthomolecular Psychiatry, Karpat Publishing Company, Cleveland, Ohio, 44101, 1971.

Recommended Dietary Allowances, National Academy of Sciences, National Research Council, Washington, D.C., 1968.

Sandler, Benjamin P., *How to Prevent Heart Attacks*, Lee Foundation for Nutritional Research, Milwaukee, Wisconsin, 1958.

Steincrohn, Peter J., M.D., *The Most Common Misdiagnosed Disease: Low Blood Sugar*, Henry Regnery Company, Chicago, 1972.

Stone, Irwin, *The Healing Factor, Vitamin C Against Disease*, Grosset and Dunlap, New York, 1972.

Szent-Györgyi, Albert, *The Living State*, The Academic Press, New York, 1972.

Williams, Roger J., *Nutrition Against Disease*, Pitman Publishing Corporation, New York, 1971.

Yudkin, John, *Sweet and Dangerous*, Peter H. Wyden, Inc., New York, 1972

Where Megavitamin Therapy and/or Information Are Available

ALABAMA

Birmingham 35223
ALABAMA CHAPTER,
American Schizophrenia Association
Mr. Glenn Ireland, II
P.O. Box 7497
Phone: 205-853-9780

CALIFORNIA

Fair Oaks 95628
SACRAMENTO CHAPTER,
American Schizophrenia Association
Ms. Evelyn M. Robison
5821 Hoffman Lane
Phone: 916-967-1411

Garden Grove 92641
ORANGE COUNTY CHAPTER,
American Schizophrenia Association
Mr. Robert Claar
P.O. Box 1191
Phone: 714-543-5470

Hollywood 90028
LOS ANGELES CHAPTER,
American Schizophrenia Association
Mr. Joseph DeSilva
P.O. Box 1776
Phone: 213-487-7070

Los Angeles 90069
Harvey Ross, M.D.
9201 Sunset Blvd.

Oakland 94604
ALAMEDA COUNTY CHAPTER,
American Schizophrenia Association
Mr. Walter B. King
P.O. Box 1484
Phone: 415-523-3864

Orinda 94563
MT. DIABLO CHAPTER,
American Schizophrenia Association
Mr. Jack Brannan
9 Corte Bombera
Phones: 415-254-6090; 415-935-3152

San Francisco
SAN FRANCISCO CHAPTER,
American Schizophrenia Association
2037 Irving St., Room 212
Phone: 415-681-1140

Santa Monica 90403
Granville F. Knight, M.D.
2901 Wilshire Blvd., Suite 345

Stanford 94305
Linus Pauling
Professor of Chemistry
Stanford University

CONNECTICUT

Avon 06001
CONNECTICUT CHAPTER,
American Schizophrenia Association
Judith J. Haines
68 Old Wood Road
Phone: 203-673-5820

Green Farms 06436

Fairfield County Chapter,
Huxley Institute Chapter
Fairfield County
Phones: 203-227-2192; 203-227-1847

DISTRICT OF COLUMBIA

Washington, D. C. Chapter,
American Schizophrenia Association
The Computer Building
11141 Georgia Ave., Suite 224
Wheaton, Md. 20902
Phone: 301-949-8282

FLORIDA

Key West

Dr. Moke W. Williams
1029 Catherine St.

ILLINOIS

Chicago

Illinois Chapter,
American Schizophrenia Association
Mr. Robert J. Burdett
Bankers Bldg., Suite 2220
105 West Adams St.
Phone: 312-798-2367

IOWA

Cedar Rapids 52406

Iowa Chapter,
American Schizophrenia Association
Mr. Jack Rector
Box 535
Phones: North Iowa (319-547-2683); Central Iowa (515-448-4410); East Iowa (319-364-0524)

256

MAINE

Brunswick 04011
Maine Chapter,
American Schizophrenia Association
Pine Tree Schiz. Fdn.
Box 356
Phone: 207-942-0214

MARYLAND

Frederick 21071
Noland D. C. Lewis, M.D.
Route 5

Towson 21204
Baltimore Chapter,
American Schizophrenia Association
Mrs. Georgiana Reiblich
7020 Charles Ridge Road
Phones: 301-823-8373; 301-828-4542

MASSACHUSETTS

Boston
Mark D. Altschule, M.D.
Harvard Medical School

South Attleboro
W. H. Philpott, M.D.
Fuller Memorial Hospital

MICHIGAN

Allen Park 48101
W. E. Beebe, M.D.
7636 Allen Road

Detroit 48236
Schizophrenia Foundation of Michigan
P.O. Box 5267

MINNESOTA

Minneapolis 55435
MINNESOTA CHAPTER,
American Schizophrenia Association
Mrs. Ella Mae Richey
6950 France Ave., S., Room 14
Phone: 612-922-6916

MISSOURI

Clayton 63105
Dr. Robert Deitchman
The Oxford Building
141 N. Meramic Ave.

St. Louis 63130
Marijan Herjanic, M.D.
Department of Psychiatry
Washington University

St. Louis
Amedeo S. Marrazzi, M.D.
University of Missouri Medical School, Institute of Psychiatry

St. Louis
MISSOURI CHAPTER,
American Schizophrenia Association
Mrs. John Lehmann
10 Apple Tree Lane
Phone: 314-993-0685

NEVADA

Reno
F. W. Allport, M.D.
674 N. Arlington St.

NEW JERSEY

Montclair 07043
Theodore Robie, M.D.
1 Upper Mountain Avenue

Skillman 08558

NEW JERSEY CHAPTER,
American Schizophrenia Association
Mrs. Ann Seidler
c/o Box 25
Phone: 201-375-0809

Skillman 08558

Carl C. Pfeiffer, M.D.
c/o Box 25

Trenton 06818

Jack Ward, M.D.
333 W. State St.

NEW YORK

Eastchester 10709

HUXLEY WESTCHESTER CHAPTER,
Mrs. Betty Plante
1209 California Road
Phones: 914-337-2252; 914-668-3943; 914-693-0173

Manhasset, L. I. 11030

David R. Hawkins, M.D.
The North Nassau Mental Health Center
1691 Northern Blvd.

Manhasset, L. I. 11030

LONG ISLAND CHAPTER,
American Schizophrenia Association
The North Nassau Mental Health Center
1691 Northern Blvd.
Phone: 516-365-8597

New York City

American Schizophrenia Association
(Same address as Huxley Institute, N.Y.C.)

New York City

Dr. Harold Rosenberg
270 West End Avenue

New York City 10016

A. Allan Cott, M.D.
303 Lexington Ave.

New York City
Fryer Research Center
345 W. 58th St.

New York City 10036
Huxley Institute for Biosocial Research (National Office)
1114 First Avenue
New York City
Phone: 972-0705

New York City
H. L. Newbold, M.D.
Suite 19N, 251 E. 51st St.

New York City 10003
NEW YORK CITY CHAPTER,
American Schizophrenia Association
Clinic 265-5805
Mrs. Douglas Fryer
15 Gramercy Park
Phone: 212-254-7919

Rochester
Leo G. Abood, Ph.D.
University of Rochester
Center for Brain Research

NORTH CAROLINA

Charlotte 28205
NORTH CAROLINA CHAPTER,
American Schizophrenia Association
Mrs. Arthur Newcombe.
3101 Loma Lane

Reidsville 27320
Frederick R. Klenner, M.D., F.C.C.P.
217 Gilmer St.

OHIO

Mayfield Heights 44124
OHIO CHAPTER,
American Schizophrenia Association
Mr. Chester Hicks
6028 Mayfield Road

260

PENNSYLVANIA

Philadelphia 19129
Charles Shagass, M.D.
Eastern Pennsylvania Psychiatric Institute

Philadelphia
Ralph A. Shaw, M.D.
Hahnemann Medical College and Hospital
230 N. Broad

VIRGINIA

Virginia Beach 23452
VIRGINIA CHAPTER,
American Schizophrenia Association
Mrs. Sam B. Ferrell, Jr.
Box 2342
Phone: 703-486-3983

WASHINGTON

Seattle 98122
SEATTLE CHAPTER,
American Schizophrenia Association
Mr. Alex R. Jancewicz
1414 E. Union St.
Phone: 206-325-6542

WISCONSIN

Eau Claire 54701
Joseph M. Tobin, M.D.
Northwest Psychiatric Clinic Research Center
605 Walker Ave.

Kenosha 53140
WISCONSIN CHAPTER,
American Schizophrenia Association
Mrs. L. Sanders
8917 24th Ave.
Phone: 414-694-5062

ARGENTINA

Edmundo Fischer, M.D.
National University
Buenos Aires, Argentina

Jose Yaryura-Tobias, M.D.
Rioja 3417
La Lucilla (P.B.A.), Argentina

BOLIVIA

BOLIVIA FOUNDATION
J. Ribero Mendez
Casilla 370
Cochabama, Bolivia

CANADA

T. Wechowich, M.D.
Edmonton, Alberta

M. Galambos, M.D.
Crease Clinic
Essondale, British Columbia

Donald C. MacDonald, M.D.
Hollywood Psychiatric Hospital
515 Fifth Ave.
New Westminster, British Columbia

J. Ross MacLean, M.D.
Hollywood Psychiatric Hospital
515 Fifth Ave.
New Westminster, British Columbia

R. Glen Green, M.D., C.M.
301 Medical Building
Prince Albert, Saskatchewan

CANADIAN FOUNDATION
Mr. I. J. Kahan
#10—1630 Albert St.
Regina, Saskatchewan
Phone: 306-527-7969

Abram Hoffer, M.D., Ph.D., President
Huxley Institute for Biosocial Research (in New York)
1201 CN Towers
First Avenue South
Saskatoon, Saskatchewan

Bella Kowalson, M.D.
Kobrinsky Clinic
208 Edmonton St.
Winnipeg, Manitoba

ENGLAND

GREAT BRITAIN FOUNDATION
Mrs. Gwynneth Hemmings
Llanfair Hall
Caernarvon, England

Index

264

Boston University Medical Center, 236
Boyd, Alan, 20
Boyle, Dr. Edwin, 143
Brain, damage to, 50, 59, 80, 148, 172, 200, 219, 220
Breakfast, importance of, 5, 11, 14, 59, 62, 132, 162, 194
Briggs, Dr. George M., 123
Briggs, Dr. Michael H., 161
Brighton Hospital, Detroit, 55
British Medical Journal, 18, 59, 161, 243
Bronchitis, 243
Butler, Dr. Frank S., 39

C

Caesar, Sid, 215
Caffeine (see also "Coffee"), 96, 194, 208, 238
Calcium, 50, 117, 118
California State University, Fullerton, 22
California, University of, 57, 58, 235
Calories, 42 ff., 46, 58, 60, 61, 78, 211
Campbell, Dr. Robert J., 33
Canada, 62, 66, 108, 249
Canadian Medical Journal, 165
Canadian Schizophrenia Foundation, 158, 160
Cancer, 44, 117, 162, 243, 244
Capistrano-by-the-Sea Neuropsychiatric Hospital, 155
Carbohydrates, 60, 131, 134, 178, 185, 191, 195, 197, 201, 202, 212, 230

Carbohydrates, refined, 8, 36, 39, 159, 173, 213, 219
Caroline Institute, Stockholm, 67
Chafetz, Dr. Morris E., 77
Chelating agents, 118
Cheraskin, Dr. E., 54
Cherubin, Charles, 124
Chicago Alcoholic Treatment Center, 77
Chicago Tribune, 76
Child abuse cases, 91
Children addicted to drugs, 98, 109
Children, drinking and drug problems among, 71 ff., 96
Children, hyperactive, 79, 107, 140, 165 ff., 219
Children, hyperactive, treatment of, 167, 170, 176, 178, 183
Children, poor eating habits of, 130 ff., 169, 219
Chloromycetin, 118
Cholesterol, 52, 69, 116, 119, 143, 144
Christakis, Dr. George, 50
Chromium, 174, 185, 186
Chromosomes, 66
Cigarette consumption, 240
Cigarettes (see also "Smoking"), 12, 58, 88, 133, 194, 208
Cigars, 242, 246
Circulation, improvement of, 52
Cirrhosis of liver, 44, 55, 60, 63, 68, 197
Coca-Cola, 79, 127
Cocaine, 78, 79, 228
Coca leaves, 78, 228
Cocktail parties, 15

MEGAVITAMIN THERAPY

FOOD AND NUTRITION BOARD, NATIONAL ACADEMY OF SCIENCES—NATIONAL RESEARCH COUNCIL RECOMMENDED DAILY DIETARY ALLOWANCES,[a] Revised 1968
Designed for the maintenance of good nutrition of practically all healthy people in the U.S.A.

FAT-SOLUBLE VITAMINS

AGE [b] (years) From	Up to	WEIGHT (kg)	(lbs)	HEIGHT cm	(in.)	kcal	PROTEIN (gm)	VITAMIN A ACTIVITY (IU)	VITAMIN D (IU)	VITAMIN E ACTIVITY (IU)
Infants										
0–1/6		4	9	55	22	kg X 120	kg X 2.2[e]	1,500	400	5
1/6–1/2		7	15	63	25	kg X 110	kg X 2.0[e]	1,500	400	5
1/2–1		9	20	72	28	kg X 100	kg X 1.8[e]	1,500	400	5
Children										
1–2		12	26	81	32	1,100	25	2,000	400	10
2–3		14	31	91	36	1,250	25	2,000	400	10
3–4		16	35	100	39	1,400	30	2,500	400	10
4–6		19	42	110	43	1,600	30	2,500	400	10
6–8		23	51	121	48	2,000	35	3,500	400	15
8–10		28	62	131	52	2,200	40	3,500	400	15
Males										
10–12		35	77	140	55	2,500	45	4,500	400	20
12–14		43	95	151	59	2,700	50	5,000	400	20
14–18		59	130	170	67	3,000	60	5,000	400	25
18–22		67	147	175	69	2,800	60	5,000	400	30
22–35		70	154	175	69	2,800	65	5,000	–	30
35–55		70	154	173	68	2,600	65	5,000	–	30
50–75+		70	154	171	67	2,400	65	5,000	–	30
Females										
10–12		35	77	142	56	2,250	50	4,500	400	20
12–14		44	97	154	61	2,300	50	5,000	400	20
14–16		52	114	157	62	2,400	55	5,000	400	25
16–18		54	119	160	63	2,300	55	5,000	400	25
18–22		58	128	163	64	2,000	55	5,000	400	25
22–35		58	128	163	64	2,000	55	5,000	–	25
35–55		58	128	160	63	1,850	55	5,000	–	25
55–75+		58	128	157	62	1,700	55	5,000	–	25
Pregnancy						+200	65	6,000	400	30
Lactation						+1,000	75	8,000	400	30

a The allowance levels are intended to cover individual variations among most normal persons as they live in the United States under usual environmental stresses. The recommended allowances can be attained with a variety of common foods, providing other nutrients for which human requirements have been less well defined. See text for more-detailed discussion of allowances and of nutrients not tabulated.

b Entries on lines for age range 22-35 years represent the reference man and woman at age 22. All other entries represent allowances for the midpoint of the specified age range.

WATER-SOLUBLE VITAMINS							MINERALS				
ASCORBIC ACID (mg)	FOLACIN c (mg)	NIACIN d (mg equiv)	RIBOFLAVIN (mg)	THIAMIN (mg)	VITAMIN B6 (mg)	VITAMIN B12 (µg)	CALCIUM (g)	PHOSPHORUS (g)	IODINE (µg)	IRON (mg)	MAGNESIUM (mg)
35	0.05	5	0.4	0.2	0.2	1.0	0.4	0.2	25	6	40
35	0.05	7	0.5	0.4	0.3	1.5	0.5	0.4	40	10	60
35	0.1	8	0.6	0.5	0.4	2.0	0.6	0.5	45	15	70
40	0.1	8	0.6	0.6	0.5	2.0	0.7	0.7	55	15	100
40	0.2	8	0.7	0.6	0.6	2.5	0.8	0.8	60	15	150
40	0.2	9	0.8	0.7	0.7	3	0.8	0.8	70	10	200
40	0.2	11	0.9	0.8	0.9	4	0.8	0.8	80	10	200
40	0.2	13	1.1	1.0	1.0	4	0.9	0.9	100	10	250
40	0.3	15	1.2	1.1	1.2	5	1.0	1.0	110	10	250
40	0.4	17	1.3	1.3	1.4	5	1.2	1.2	125	10	300
45	0.4	18	1.4	1.4	1.6	5	1.4	1.4	135	18	350
55	0.4	20	1.5	1.5	1.8	5	1.4	1.4	150	18	400
60	0.4	18	1.6	1.4	2.0	5	0.8	0.8	140	10	400
60	0.4	18	1.7	1.4	2.0	5	0.8	0.8	140	10	350
60	0.4	17	1.7	1.3	2.0	5	0.8	0.8	125	10	350
60	0.4	14	1.7	1.2	2.0	6	0.8	0.8	110	10	350
40	0.4	15	1.3	1.1	1.4	5	1.2	1.2	110	18	300
45	0.4	15	1.4	1.2	1.6	5	1.3	1.3	115	18	350
50	0.4	16	1.4	1.2	1.8	5	1.3	1.3	120	18	350
50	0.4	15	1.5	1.2	2.0	5	1.3	1.3	115	18	350
55	0.4	13	1.5	1.0	2.0	5	0.8	0.8	100	18	350
55	0.4	13	1.5	1.0	2.0	5	0.8	0.8	100	18	300
55	0.4	13	1.5	1.0	2.0	5	0.8	0.8	90	18	300
55	0.4	13	1.5	1.0	2.0	6	0.8	0.8	80	10	300
60	0.8	15	1.8	+0.1	2.5	8	+0.4	+0.4	125	18	450
60	0.5	20	2.0	+0.5	2.5	6	+0.5	+0.5	150	18	450

c The folacin allowances refer to dietary sources as determined by *Lactobacillus casei* assay. Pure forms of folacin may be effective in doses less than ¼ of the RDA.

d Niacin equivalents include dietary sources of the vitamin itself plus 1 mg equivalent for each 60 mg of dietary tryptophan.

e Assumes protein equivalent to human milk. For proteins not 100 percent utilized factors should be increased propotionately.

The Best Books on Health
LARCHMONT BOOKS

All You Should Know about Arthritis by Ruth Adams and Frank Murray. *What Adams and Murray have to say about arthritis.* 256 pages, $2.25.

Almonds to Zoybeans by "Mothey" Parsons. *The A to Z cookbook of quality protein meals without meat.* 192 pages, $1.50.

Beverages by Adams and Murray. *The advantages of choosing healthful beverages are the focus of this interesting book.* 288 pages, $1.75.

Body, Mind and the B Vitamins by Adams and Murray. *The most informative book ever written about the B vitamins and their essential role in mental and physical health.* 320 pages, $1.95.

The Compleat Herbal by Ben Charles Harris. *An authentic, comprehensive guide to medicinal plants and herbs.* 248 pages, $1.95.

The Complete Home Guide to All the Vitamins by Ruth Adams. *This popular and valuable home reference answers all your questions about vitamins.* 432 pages, $2.75

Eating in Eden by Ruth Adams. *Learn to appreciate the joys and benefits of natural foods.* 206 pages, $1.75.

Fighting Depression by Harvey Ross, M.D. *This book contains valuable material for anyone suffering from depression.* 224 pages, $1.95.

Food for Beauty by Helena Rubenstein. *Frank Murray has revised and updated Miss Rubenstein's 1938 classic on diet and beauty.* 256 pages, $1.95.

The Good Seeds, the Rich Grains, the Hardy Nuts for a Happier, Healthier Life by Adams and Murray. *This book cracks all the myths about the value of over-processed foods.* 352 pages, $1.75.

Health Foods by Adams and Murray. *This complete mini-encyclopedia tells all about health foods.* 352 pages, $2.50.

How to Control Your Allergies by Robert Forman, Ph.D. *Helps you find out which chemical or natural allergen is causing discomfort and how to live healthfully with an allergy.* 256 pages, $1.95.

Is Low Blood Sugar Making You a Nutritional Cripple? by Adams and Murray. *The latest information about hypoglycemia, including the proper diet and supplements.* 176 pages, $1.75.

Lose Weight, Feel Great! by John Yudkin, M.D., Ph.D. *This book describes the healthful diet for those who want to lose pounds and inches permanently.* 220 pages. $1.75.

Megavitamin Therapy by Adams and Murray. *Describes this great breakthrough in treatment for alcoholics, schizophrenics, drug addicts, and hyperactive children.* 286 pages, *$2.25.*

Minerals: Kill or Cure? by Adams and Murray. *The first complete book ever written about minerals and their essential place in a healthful diet.* 368 pages, $1.95.

The New High Fiber Diet by Adams and Murray. *This book contains important information on the value of fiber in your diet and includes over 250 delicious high fiber recipes.* 320 pages. $2.25.

Program Your Heart for Health by Frank Murray. *One of the most current books on the role of proper nutrition in preventing heart attack or stroke. Valuable information on a vital subject.* 368 pages, $2.95.

Have you read the important
LARCHMONT BOOKS
on this and the preceding page?

*They are available at your local
health and natural foods store.*